INSTRUCTIONS

1. Lay the tortillas or wraps out on a flat surface.

2. Spread 1/2 tbsp of mayonnaise or Greek yogurt onto each wrap.

3. Layer the turkey slices, avocado slices, lettuce, and tomato slices onto the center of each wrap.

4. Season with salt and pepper.

5. Fold the bottom of the wrap up over the filling, then fold in the sides and continue rolling up tightly into a wrap.

6. Cut the wraps in half diagonally to serve.

Tips:
• Use whole grain tortillas or wraps for added fiber.

• Swap out the turkey for grilled chicken or roast beef if preferred.

• Add other veggies like shredded carrots, cucumber, or sprouts.

• Use hummus or guacamole instead of mayo/yogurt for a healthier spread.

• Serve with baked chips, carrot sticks, or a side salad for a complete lunch.

This turkey and avocado wrap is packed with protein, healthy fats, and fresh veggies • perfect for refueling hungry teenage boys!

INGREDIENTS

- 1 bunch kale, washed and dried thoroughly
- 1-2 tablespoons olive oil
- 1/2 teaspoon sea salt

Optional Seasonings:
- 1/4 teaspoon garlic powder
- 1/4 teaspoon onion powder
- 1/4 teaspoon paprika
- 1/4 teaspoon cayenne pepper

2. Kale chips

INSTRUCTIONS

1. Preheat your oven to 400°F (200°C).

2. Line a baking sheet with parchment paper or foil.

3. Place the salmon fillets on the prepared baking sheet.

4. In a small bowl, mix together the olive oil, lemon juice, garlic powder, and dried dill.

5. Brush the salmon fillets with the oil and seasoning mixture, making sure to coat the tops and sides.

6. Season with salt and pepper to taste.

7. Bake the salmon for 12•15 minutes, or until it flakes easily with a fork and reaches an internal temperature of 145°F (63°C).

8. Serve the baked salmon immediately, garnished with lemon wedges if desired.

Tips:
• For extra flavor, you can also add a sprinkle of paprika or cayenne pepper.

• Serve the baked salmon with roasted vegetables, a side salad, or steamed rice for a complete and balanced meal.

• Leftovers can be used in salads, wraps, or pasta dishes throughout the week.

This baked salmon recipe is quick, easy, and packed with healthy omega•3 fatty acids • perfect for growing teenage boys!

INGREDIENTS

- 1 head of broccoli, cut into florets
- 1-2 tablespoons water
- Salt and pepper to taste

Optional Additions:
- 1 tablespoon lemon juice
- 1 tablespoon olive oil
- 1 clove garlic, minced
- 2 tablespoons grated Parmesan cheese

3. Steamed broccoli

In today's fast-paced world, where convenience often trumps nutrition, many men find themselves facing health challenges that can be mitigated or even reversed with the right dietary choices. One such challenge is fatty liver disease, a condition that affects millions of people worldwide and is closely linked to diet and lifestyle. *"Fatty Liver Cookbook for Men: 115+ Delicious Recipes for Fatty Liver. 60 Day Meal Detox and Cleanse Your Liver"* is crafted to address this critical issue head-on, offering practical solutions and tasty recipes to help you take charge of your liver health.

Why This Cookbook?

This cookbook is specifically designed for men who want to improve their liver health through nutritious and satisfying meals. It's not just a collection of recipes but a comprehensive guide that integrates dietary changes into your daily life. By following the recipes and meal plans in this book, you will embark on a 60-day journey to detoxify and cleanse your liver, setting the stage for long-term health and wellness.

Understanding Fatty Liver Disease

Before diving into the recipes, it's essential to understand what fatty liver disease is and why it's crucial to address it. Fatty liver disease occurs when excess fat builds up in the liver cells, leading to inflammation and potential liver damage. This book explains the causes, symptoms, and risks associated with fatty liver disease and highlights the vital role that diet plays in managing and reversing this condition.

The Power of Nutrition

A liver-friendly diet focuses on whole, unprocessed foods that provide essential nutrients while avoiding those that can harm the liver. This cookbook emphasizes the importance of fruits, vegetables, lean proteins, whole grains, and healthy fats, offering recipes that are not only good for your liver but also delicious and easy to prepare.

What's Inside?

- *115+ Delicious Recipes:* From hearty breakfasts and satisfying lunches to healing dinners and smart snacks, this book provides a wide variety of recipes that cater to different tastes and dietary preferences. Each recipe is crafted to support liver health without compromising on flavor.

- *60 Day Meal Plan:* A detailed meal plan helps you detox and cleanse your liver over two months. This structured approach ensures you get the right balance of nutrients and makes it easier to stick to a liver-friendly diet.

- *Practical Tips and Advice:* Learn how to make healthier food choices, plan your meals, and maintain a liver-friendly lifestyle. The book offers practical advice on grocery shopping, kitchen organization, and cooking techniques that simplify the process of eating well.

Embarking on a liver-friendly diet doesn't mean sacrificing flavor or enjoyment. With "Fatty Liver Cookbook for Men," you'll discover that healthy eating can be both delicious and fulfilling. This book is your companion on the path to better liver health, providing you with the knowledge, tools, and recipes you need to make lasting changes. Here's to a healthier liver and a healthier you!

INSTRUCTIONS

1. Preheat grill to medium•high heat.

2. In a shallow dish, combine the olive oil, garlic powder, onion powder, paprika, oregano, salt, and pepper. Add the chicken breasts and turn to coat both sides.

3. Grill the chicken for 5•7 minutes per side, or until the internal temperature reaches 165°F.

4. Let the chicken rest for 5 minutes before serving.

Tips:
• Serve with grilled veggies, a baked potato, or a fresh salad for a complete meal.

• Marinate the chicken in the spice mixture for 30 minutes before grilling for extra flavor.

• Try different seasoning blends like Cajun, lemon pepper, or Italian to change up the flavor.

• Slice the grilled chicken and use it in wraps, salads, or pasta dishes.

This simple grilled chicken is packed with protein, easy to make, and sure to be a hit with hungry teenage boys!

INGREDIENTS

- 6 cups fresh spinach leaves, washed and dried
- 1/2 cup sliced mushrooms
- 1/4 cup sliced red onion
- 2 hard boiled eggs, chopped
- 2 tablespoons crumbled bacon (optional)
- 2 tablespoons toasted slivered almonds (optional)

Dressing:
- 2 tablespoons olive oil
- 1 tablespoon balsamic vinegar
- 1 teaspoon Dijon mustard
- 1 teaspoon honey
- Salt and pepper to taste

1. Spinach salad

1. Cook the quinoa according to package instructions. Fluff with a fork and set aside.

2. In a large bowl, combine the cooked quinoa, black beans, tomatoes, avocado, corn, red onion, and cilantro (if using).

3. Drizzle the lime juice over the top and sprinkle with cumin, chili powder, salt, and pepper. Gently toss to combine.

4. Serve the quinoa and black bean bowl warm or chilled.

Tips:
• For extra protein, top with grilled chicken or shrimp.
• Add other veggies like bell peppers, spinach, or roasted sweet potatoes.

• Customize the seasonings to your taste • try adding garlic powder, paprika, or cayenne.

• Serve with tortilla chips, salsa, or a dollop of Greek yogurt on the side.

• This recipe can be easily doubled or tripled to meal prep for the week.

This quinoa and black bean bowl is packed with fiber, protein, and healthy fats • perfect for fueling growing teenage boys!

INGREDIENTS

- 1 lb fresh asparagus, trimmed
- 2 tablespoons olive oil
- 1 teaspoon lemon zest
- 1 tablespoon lemon juice
- 1/2 teaspoon salt
- 1/4 teaspoon black pepper

4. Grilled asparagus

1. In a clear glass or jar, layer the ingredients in the following order:
  • 1/4 cup Greek yogurt
  • 1/4 cup fresh berries
  • 2 tbsp granola or toasted oats
  • Repeat the layers until you reach the top of the glass/jar.

2. If desired, drizzle 1 tsp of honey over the top of the parfait.

3. Refrigerate until ready to serve.

Tips:
• Use a variety of berries for different colors and flavors.

• Swap out the granola for crushed nuts, chia seeds, or shredded coconut.

• Add a sprinkle of cinnamon or vanilla extract for extra flavor.

• Make these parfaits in advance for a quick and easy breakfast or snack.

• Serve in individual glasses or jars for a fun, portable option.

This Greek yogurt parfait is a nutritious and delicious option for teenage boys. The combination of protein•rich yogurt, fiber•filled berries, and crunchy granola makes it a satisfying and energizing treat.

INGREDIENTS

- 1 lb Brussels sprouts, trimmed and halved
- 2 tablespoons olive oil
- 1 teaspoon garlic powder
- 1 teaspoon paprika
- 1/2 teaspoon salt
- 1/4 teaspoon black pepper

5. Roasted Brussels sprouts

INSTRUCTIONS

1. Heat the 2 tbsp of vegetable or sesame oil in a large skillet or wok over high heat.

2. Add the chicken and stir•fry for 3•4 minutes until lightly browned.

3. Add the garlic and ginger and stir•fry for 1 minute until fragrant.

4. Add the bell pepper, broccoli, mushrooms, and snow peas. Stir•fry for 4•5 minutes until the vegetables are tender•crisp.

5. In a small bowl, whisk together the soy sauce, rice vinegar/lime juice, and 1 tsp sesame oil.

6. Pour the sauce into the skillet and toss everything together until well coated.

7. Season with salt and pepper to taste.

8. Serve the stir•fry immediately over cooked brown rice or quinoa.

Tips:
• Use a variety of colorful vegetables like carrots, zucchini, or bok choy.
• Swap the chicken for tofu or shrimp for a different protein option.
• Add a sprinkle of crushed red pepper flakes for a little heat.
• Serve with steamed edamame or a side salad for a complete meal.

This veggie•packed stir•fry is a great way to get teenage boys to eat their greens! The combination of tender chicken, crisp veggies, and flavorful sauce makes it a delicious and nutritious meal.

INGREDIENTS

- 1 head of cauliflower, cut into florets
- 1 tablespoon olive oil
- 1 clove garlic, minced
- 1/4 teaspoon salt
- 1/8 teaspoon black pepper

6. Cauliflower rice

1. Bring a large pot of salted water to a boil. Cook the whole grain pasta according to package instructions until al dente. Drain and set aside.

2. In a large skillet, heat the olive oil over medium heat. Add the diced onion and sauté for 3•4 minutes until translucent.

3. Add the minced garlic and sauté for 1 minute until fragrant.

4. Pour in the can of crushed tomatoes and stir in the tomato paste. Season with the dried oregano, basil, salt, and pepper.

5. Simmer the tomato sauce for 10•15 minutes, stirring occasionally, until thickened slightly.

6. Add the cooked whole grain pasta to the sauce and toss to coat evenly.

7. Serve the pasta warm, topped with a sprinkle of grated Parmesan cheese if desired.

Tips:
• Use a variety of whole grain pasta shapes like penne, fusilli, or spaghetti.
• For extra protein, add cooked ground turkey or Italian sausage to the sauce.
• Sneak in extra veggies by sautéing diced zucchini, bell peppers, or spinach with the onions.
• Serve with a side salad or garlic bread for a complete meal.
• Leftovers reheat well for easy lunches or dinners throughout the week.

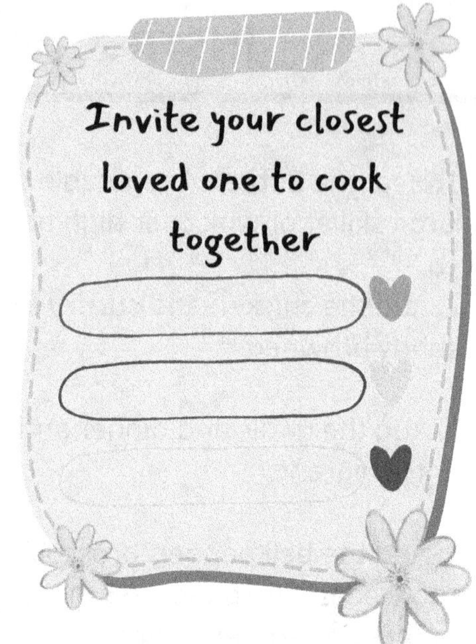

INGREDIENTS

- 4-5 medium carrots, peeled and cut into sticks
- 1 cup homemade or store-bought hummus

For the Homemade Hummus:
- 1 (15 oz) can chickpeas, drained and rinsed
- 2 tablespoons tahini
- 2 tablespoons lemon juice
- 1 clove garlic, minced
- 2 tablespoons olive oil
- 1/4 teaspoon ground cumin
- 1/4 teaspoon salt
- 2-3 tablespoons water (if needed to blend)

7. Carrot sticks with hummus

INSTRUCTIONS

1. In a large bowl, gently mix together the ground beef, garlic powder, onion powder, Worcestershire sauce, salt, and pepper until just combined. Be careful not to overmix.

2. Divide the beef mixture into 4 equal portions and shape them into patties, each about 4•5 inches wide and 1/2 inch thick.

3. Preheat your grill or a large skillet over medium•high heat.

4. Cook the burgers for 3•4 minutes per side, or until they reach your desired level of doneness. The internal temperature should reach 160°F for food safety.

5. Toast the whole wheat buns while the burgers are cooking.

6. Place the cooked burgers on the toasted buns and top with your desired toppings.

Tips:
• Use lean ground beef to keep the burgers healthier and lower in fat.
• Experiment with different seasonings like chili powder, cumin, or smoked paprika.
• Serve the burgers with baked sweet potato fries or a fresh salad for a complete meal.
• Make a double batch and freeze the uncooked patties for easy meal prep.
• Encourage teens to get creative with their burger toppings!

INGREDIENTS

- 1 large cucumber, sliced into thin rounds
- 1 tablespoon apple cider vinegar
- 1 teaspoon honey
- 1/2 teaspoon dried dill (or 1 tablespoon fresh dill)
- 1/4 teaspoon salt
- 1/8 teaspoon black pepper

8. Cucumber slices

INSTRUCTIONS

1. Preheat your grill or grill pan to medium•high heat.

2. In a large bowl, toss the chopped vegetables with the olive oil, oregano, garlic powder, salt, and pepper until evenly coated.

3. Thread the vegetables onto the skewers, alternating the different types.

4. Grill the vegetable skewers for 12•15 minutes, turning occasionally, until the vegetables are tender and lightly charred.

5. Serve the grilled vegetable skewers hot, alongside grilled chicken, steak, or tofu for a complete meal.

Tips:
• Use a variety of colorful vegetables like cherry tomatoes, eggplant, or asparagus.
• Soak wooden skewers in water for 30 minutes before using to prevent them from burning.
• Brush the skewers with a bit of balsamic glaze or teriyaki sauce for extra flavor.
• Serve the grilled veggies over a bed of quinoa or brown rice for a heartier dish.
• Encourage teens to get creative and customize their skewers with their favorite veggies.

These grilled vegetable skewers are a fun and delicious way to get teenage boys to eat more plant•based foods. The combination of tender, flavorful veggies makes for a satisfying and nutritious side or main dish.

INGREDIENTS

- 3-4 medium zucchini, spiralized or julienned into noodle-like strips
- 1 tablespoon olive oil
- 2 cloves garlic, minced
- 1/4 teaspoon red pepper flakes (optional)
- 1/4 cup grated Parmesan cheese (optional)
- Salt and black pepper to taste

1. Preheat your oven to 400°F (200°C). Line a large baking sheet with parchment paper.

2. In a large bowl, toss the sweet potato fry shapes with the olive oil, paprika, garlic powder, salt, and pepper until evenly coated.

3. Spread the seasoned sweet potato fries in a single layer on the prepared baking sheet, making sure they are not touching each other.

4. Bake for 20•25 minutes, flipping the fries halfway through, until they are tender and lightly browned.

5. Remove the baked sweet potato fries from the oven and serve hot.

Tips:
• For crispier fries, spread the fries out in a single layer and avoid overcrowding the baking sheet.
• Try different seasoning blends like chili powder, cumin, or cajun spice.
• Serve the baked sweet potato fries with a side of ranch, honey mustard, or ketchup for dipping.
• Experiment with different cut shapes like wedges or tater tot•style bites.
• Leftovers can be reheated in the oven or air fryer for a quick and easy snack.

These baked sweet potato fries are a healthier alternative to traditional french fries, but still packed with flavor that teenage boys are sure to love. The combination of natural sweetness and savory spices makes them irresistible.

INGREDIENTS

- 4 bell peppers (any color), halved lengthwise and seeds removed
- 1 lb ground turkey or lean ground beef
- 1 cup cooked brown rice
- 1 small onion, diced
- 3 cloves garlic, minced
- 1 (15 oz) can diced tomatoes
- 1 teaspoon dried oregano
- 1/2 teaspoon dried basil
- 1/4 teaspoon red pepper flakes (optional)
- 1 cup shredded mozzarella cheese
- Salt and black pepper to taste

INSTRUCTIONS

1. In a medium bowl, combine the drained tuna, Greek yogurt, mayonnaise, Dijon mustard, celery, red onion, and parsley (if using). Mix well until fully incorporated.

2. Season the tuna salad with salt and pepper to taste.

3. Spread the tuna salad evenly onto 4 slices of the whole grain bread.

4. Top each tuna salad•covered slice with another slice of bread to create 4 sandwiches.

5. Serve the tuna salad sandwiches immediately, or wrap them individually and refrigerate until ready to eat.

Tips:
• For extra crunch, add chopped dill pickles or toasted walnuts to the tuna salad.
• Swap out the Greek yogurt for mashed avocado for a creamy, healthy alternative.
• Use a variety of whole grain breads like whole wheat, rye, or multigrain.
• Serve the tuna salad sandwiches with a side of carrot sticks, apple slices, or baked chips.
• This recipe can be easily doubled or tripled to meal prep for the week.

This tuna salad sandwich on whole grain bread is a nutritious and satisfying option for teenage boys. The combination of protein•rich tuna, fiber•filled whole grains, and fresh veggies makes it a well•balanced meal.

INGREDIENTS

- 1 lb eggplant, cut into 1-inch cubes
- 2 tablespoons olive oil
- 1 onion, sliced
- 3 cloves garlic, minced
- 1 red bell pepper, sliced
- 1 cup sliced mushrooms
- 2 tablespoons low-sodium soy sauce or tamari
- 1 tablespoon rice vinegar
- 1 teaspoon honey
- 1/4 teaspoon red pepper flakes (optional)
- Salt and black pepper to taste
- Chopped fresh parsley or basil for garnish (optional)

INSTRUCTIONS

1. In a small bowl, whisk together the eggs and milk/water until well combined. Season with a pinch of salt and pepper.

2. Heat the olive oil in a nonstick skillet over medium heat.

3. Add the diced bell pepper, onion, and mushrooms to the skillet. Sauté for 2•3 minutes until the vegetables are tender.

4. Pour the egg mixture into the skillet and let it sit for 30 seconds to a minute to set the bottom.

5. Using a spatula, gently push the cooked egg towards the center, tilting the pan to allow the uncooked egg to flow to the edges.

6. Once the bottom is set but the top is still a bit runny, sprinkle the baby spinach leaves over the top.

7. If using, sprinkle the shredded cheddar cheese over the spinach.

8. Fold the omelet in half and slide it onto a plate.

9. Serve the veggie•packed omelet immediately.

Tips:
• Customize the veggies based on your teen's preferences • try adding diced tomatoes, shredded zucchini, or chopped broccoli.
• For extra protein, add cooked crumbled bacon or diced ham.
• Serve the omelet with a side of whole grain toast or a fresh fruit salad.
• Prepare the omelet in advance and reheat for a quick and easy breakfast.

INGREDIENTS

- 1 lb fresh green beans, trimmed
- 2 tablespoons olive oil
- 1/4 cup sliced almonds
- 2 cloves garlic, minced
- 1 tablespoon lemon juice
- 1/4 teaspoon salt
- 1/8 teaspoon black pepper

12. Green beans almondine

1. Preheat your oven to 400°F (200°C). Line a baking sheet with parchment paper.

2. In a large bowl, combine the ground turkey, breadcrumbs, Parmesan cheese, egg, garlic, parsley, oregano, salt, and pepper. Mix until just combined, being careful not to overmix.

3. Scoop the turkey mixture and roll it into 1•inch meatballs, placing them on the prepared baking sheet.

4. Bake the meatballs for 18•20 minutes, or until they are cooked through and reach an internal temperature of 165°F (75°C).

5. Serve the homemade turkey meatballs warm, over whole grain pasta, in a sub sandwich, or as a standalone appetizer.

Tips:
• For extra flavor, try adding a teaspoon of Italian seasoning or a pinch of red pepper flakes to the meatball mixture.
• Swap the Parmesan cheese for shredded mozzarella or crumbled feta for a different taste.
• Bake the meatballs in advance and reheat them for a quick and easy meal.
• Serve the meatballs with a side of roasted vegetables or a fresh salad for a complete and balanced meal.
• Encourage teens to get creative and use the meatballs in different dishes, like meatball subs or meatball soup.

INGREDIENTS

- 2 large sweet potatoes, peeled and cut into 1/2-inch thick fry shapes
- 2 tablespoons olive oil
- 1 teaspoon paprika
- 1/2 teaspoon garlic powder
- 1/2 teaspoon onion powder
- 1/4 teaspoon cayenne pepper (optional)
- 1/2 teaspoon salt
- 1/4 teaspoon black pepper

13. Sweet potato fries (baked)

INSTRUCTIONS

1. In a large pot or Dutch oven, heat the olive oil over medium heat. Add the diced onion and sauté for 3•4 minutes until translucent.

2. Add the minced garlic and sauté for 1 minute until fragrant.

3. Stir in the diced carrots and celery. Cook for 5 minutes, stirring occasionally.

4. Add the rinsed lentils, broth, diced tomatoes, thyme, and oregano. Season with salt and pepper to taste.

5. Bring the soup to a boil, then reduce the heat and let it simmer for 20•25 minutes, or until the lentils are tender.

6. Taste and adjust seasoning as needed.

7. Serve the lentil and vegetable soup hot, garnished with chopped fresh parsley if desired.

Tips:
• For extra protein, add cooked diced chicken or crumbled turkey sausage.
• Swap out the vegetables based on your teen's preferences • try adding spinach, zucchini, or bell peppers.
• Serve the soup with crusty whole grain bread or a side salad for a complete meal.
• Freeze leftover portions for easy reheating on busy weeknights.

This lentil and vegetable soup is a nutritious and filling option for teenage boys. The combination of fiber•rich lentils, nutrient•dense veggies, and savory herbs makes it a wholesome and satisfying meal.

INGREDIENTS

- 1 medium butternut squash, peeled, seeded, and cubed (about 4 cups)
- 1 tablespoon olive oil
- 1 onion, diced
- 3 cloves garlic, minced
- 4 cups low-sodium vegetable or chicken broth
- 1 teaspoon ground cumin
- 1/2 teaspoon ground cinnamon
- 1/4 teaspoon ground nutmeg
- Salt and black pepper to taste
- Chopped fresh parsley or thyme for garnish (optional)

1. Preheat a large skillet or griddle over medium heat.

2. Lay 4 slices of the whole grain bread on a clean surface. Top each slice with 2 slices of turkey and 2 slices of cheese.

3. Place the remaining 4 slices of bread on top to create 4 sandwiches.

4. Spread the butter or olive oil spread on the outer sides of the sandwiches.

5. Carefully place the sandwiches in the preheated skillet or griddle. Cook for 3•4 minutes per side, or until the bread is golden brown and the cheese is melted.

6. Remove the grilled turkey and cheese sandwiches from the heat and let them cool for a minute before serving.

Tips:
• Use a variety of whole grain breads like whole wheat, sourdough, or rye for added fiber and nutrients.
• Experiment with different cheese options like provolone, pepper jack, or mozzarella.
• Add sliced tomato, avocado, or spinach for extra flavor and nutrition.
• Serve the grilled sandwiches with a side of baked potato wedges or a fresh fruit salad.
• Make a double batch and wrap the extra sandwiches individually for easy grab•and•go lunches.

INGREDIENTS

- 2 lbs ripe tomatoes, cut into wedges or halves
- 1 cup fresh basil leaves, torn or chopped
- 2 tablespoons extra-virgin olive oil
- 1 tablespoon balsamic vinegar
- 1 clove garlic, minced
- 1/4 teaspoon salt
- 1/8 teaspoon black pepper

15. Tomato and basil salad

INSTRUCTIONS

1. Preheat your oven to 400°F (200°C). Line a baking sheet with parchment paper or a silicone baking mat.

2. In a shallow bowl, combine the whole wheat breadcrumbs, Parmesan cheese, garlic powder, paprika, salt, and pepper.

3. In a separate shallow bowl, beat the egg.

4. Dip the chicken tenders into the beaten egg, allowing any excess to drip off. Then, dredge the chicken tenders in the breadcrumb mixture, pressing gently to help the coating adhere.

5. Arrange the breaded chicken tenders in a single layer on the prepared baking sheet. Lightly spray the tops of the chicken with cooking spray.

6. Bake for 15•18 minutes, flipping the chicken tenders halfway through, until they are golden brown and cooked through.

7. Serve the baked chicken tenders warm, with your teen's favorite dipping sauces like honey mustard, ranch, or barbecue sauce.

Tips:
• For extra crunch, try using panko breadcrumbs instead of regular breadcrumbs.
• Experiment with different seasoning blends, like Italian herbs or Cajun spices.
• Bake the chicken tenders in advance and reheat them for a quick and easy meal.
• Serve the chicken tenders with a side of roasted vegetables or a fresh salad for a complete and balanced meal.
• Encourage teens to get creative and use the chicken tenders in different dishes, like chicken Caesar wraps or chicken parmesan.

INGREDIENTS

- 2 medium apples, cored and sliced
- 1/4 cup natural almond butter
- 1 tablespoon honey (optional)
- 1/4 teaspoon ground cinnamon (optional)

16. Apple slices with almond butter

INSTRUCTIONS

1. Preheat your oven to 400°F (200°C).

2. Spread the tomato sauce evenly over the whole wheat pizza crust, leaving a small border around the edges.

3. Sprinkle the shredded mozzarella cheese over the sauce.

4. Top the pizza with the sliced mushrooms, diced bell peppers, diced onions, and sliced black olives (if using).

5. Sprinkle the dried oregano and garlic powder over the top, and season with salt and pepper to taste.

6. Bake the pizza for 12•15 minutes, or until the crust is golden brown and the cheese is melted and bubbly. Slice the pizza and serve it hot.

Tips:
• Use a variety of colorful vegetables like zucchini, spinach, or cherry tomatoes.
• Add cooked ground turkey or Italian sausage for extra protein.
• Experiment with different cheese options like feta, goat cheese, or shredded chicken.
• Serve the pizza with a fresh side salad or roasted vegetables for a complete meal.
• Encourage teens to get creative and customize their own pizza toppings.

This whole grain pizza with veggies is a delicious and nutritious option for teenage boys. The combination of fiber•rich crust, nutrient•dense toppings, and melted cheese makes it a satisfying and balanced meal.

INGREDIENTS

- 1 cup fresh blueberries
- 1 cup fresh strawberries, hulled and sliced
- 1 cup fresh raspberries
- 1 tbsp honey (optional)
- 1 tbsp fresh lemon juice
- 1 tsp lemon zest (optional)

17. Berries (blueberries, strawberries, raspberries)

1. Preheat your oven to 375°F (190°C). Grease a 9•inch oven•safe skillet or baking dish with nonstick cooking spray.

2. In a large bowl, whisk together the eggs, milk, oregano, garlic powder, salt, and pepper until well combined.

3. In the prepared skillet or baking dish, heat the olive oil over medium heat. Add the diced bell peppers, onions, and mushrooms. Sauté for 5•7 minutes until the vegetables are tender.

4. Add the baby spinach leaves and sauté for 1•2 minutes until wilted.

5. Pour the egg mixture over the sautéed vegetables and sprinkle the shredded cheese on top.

6. Transfer the skillet or baking dish to the preheated oven and bake for 18•22 minutes, or until the frittata is set and the cheese is melted.

7. Remove the frittata from the oven and let it cool for 5 minutes before slicing and serving.

Tips:
• Customize the vegetables based on your teen's preferences • try adding diced tomatoes, zucchini, or broccoli.
• For extra protein, add cooked crumbled bacon or diced ham.
• Serve the frittata with a side of whole grain toast or a fresh fruit salad.
• Prepare the frittata in advance and reheat for a quick and easy breakfast or lunch.

INGREDIENTS

- 2-3 oranges

18. Orange segments

1. In a medium bowl, mash the black beans with a fork or potato masher until slightly chunky.

2. Stir in the shredded cheese, salsa, cumin, chili powder, salt, and pepper until well combined.

3. Lay the whole wheat tortillas out on a clean surface. Divide the bean and cheese mixture evenly among the tortillas, placing it in the center.

4. Fold the bottom of the tortilla up over the filling, then fold in the sides and continue rolling up tightly into a burrito.

5. Heat a large skillet or griddle over medium heat. Place the burritos seam•side down in the skillet and cook for 2•3 minutes per side, or until lightly golden brown.

6. Serve the bean and cheese burritos warm, with additional salsa, guacamole, or sour cream on the side if desired.

Tips:
• For extra protein, add cooked ground turkey or shredded chicken to the bean and cheese mixture.
• Swap the black beans for pinto or refried beans.
• Use a variety of shredded cheeses like pepper jack or queso fresco.
• Add diced onions, bell peppers, or jalapeños for extra flavor and nutrition.
• Wrap the cooked burritos individually and freeze for easy reheating later.

This bean and cheese burrito is a satisfying and nutritious option for teenage boys. The combination of fiber•rich beans, melted cheese, and whole grain tortilla makes it a well•balanced meal.

INGREDIENTS

- 1 small to medium watermelon

INSTRUCTIONS

1. If using wooden skewers, soak them in water for 30 minutes to prevent them from burning.

2. In a large bowl, combine the shrimp, olive oil, lemon juice, garlic, oregano, paprika, salt, and pepper. Toss to coat the shrimp evenly.

3. Thread the marinated shrimp onto the skewers, leaving a small space between each one.

4. Preheat your grill or grill pan to medium•high heat.

5. Grill the shrimp skewers for 2•3 minutes per side, or until the shrimp are opaque and cooked through.

6. Serve the grilled shrimp skewers immediately, with lemon wedges on the side.

Tips:
• For extra flavor, try marinating the shrimp in the mixture for 30 minutes to an hour before grilling.
• Experiment with different seasoning blends, like Cajun, lemon•pepper, or garlic•herb.
• Serve the grilled shrimp skewers over a bed of rice or quinoa, or with a side of roasted vegetables.
• Soak wooden skewers in water for at least 30 minutes to prevent them from burning on the grill.
• Make a double batch and freeze the uncooked skewers for easy meal prep.

These grilled shrimp skewers are a delicious and nutritious option for teenage boys. The combination of lean protein, fresh seafood, and flavorful seasonings makes it a satisfying and well•balanced meal

INGREDIENTS

- 2 grapefruits

1. If using wooden skewers, soak them in water for 30 minutes to prevent them from burning.

2. In a large bowl, combine the cubed chicken, bell pepper pieces, onion pieces, and mushrooms. Drizzle with the olive oil and sprinkle with the oregano, garlic powder, salt, and pepper. Toss to coat the ingredients evenly.

3. Thread the marinated chicken and vegetables onto the skewers, alternating the ingredients.

4. Preheat your grill or grill pan to medium•high heat.

5. Grill the chicken and vegetable kebabs for 12•15 minutes, turning occasionally, until the chicken is cooked through and the vegetables are tender.

6. Serve the grilled chicken and vegetable kebabs immediately.

Tips:
• Use a variety of colorful vegetables like zucchini, cherry tomatoes, or pineapple chunks.
• Marinate the kebabs in a mixture of olive oil, lemon juice, and Italian seasoning for extra flavor.
• Soak wooden skewers in water for at least 30 minutes to prevent them from burning on the grill.
• Serve the kebabs over a bed of rice or quinoa, or with a side of roasted potatoes or a fresh salad.
• Make a double batch and freeze the uncooked kebabs for easy meal prep.

These chicken and vegetable kebabs are a delicious and nutritious option for teenage boys. The combination of lean protein, fresh produce, and flavorful seasonings makes it a well•balanced and satisfying meal.

INGREDIENTS

- 2 ripe pears

1. In a large pot or Dutch oven, cook the ground turkey over medium•high heat, breaking it up with a wooden spoon, until browned and cooked through, about 5•7 minutes.

2. Add the diced onion and minced garlic to the pot. Sauté for 2•3 minutes until the onion is translucent.

3. Stir in the diced red bell pepper, diced tomatoes, kidney beans, black beans, chili powder, cumin, oregano, smoked paprika, and cayenne pepper (if using). Season with salt and pepper to taste.

4. Bring the chili to a simmer and let it cook for 20•25 minutes, stirring occasionally, until the flavors have melded and the chili has thickened.

5. Serve the turkey chili hot, topped with shredded cheddar cheese, a dollop of sour cream, and chopped cilantro, if desired.

Tips:
• For extra protein, add cooked diced chicken or ground beef along with the turkey.
• Customize the spice level by adjusting the amount of chili powder and cayenne pepper.
• Serve the chili with cornbread, tortilla chips, or a side salad for a complete meal.
• Freeze leftover portions for easy reheating on busy weeknights.

This turkey chili is a hearty and nutritious option that teenage boys are sure to love. The combination of lean protein, fiber•rich beans, and bold spices makes it a satisfying and flavorful dish.

INGREDIENTS

- 1 whole pineapple

INSTRUCTIONS

1. Preheat your oven to 400°F (200°C). Line a baking sheet with parchment paper.

2. In a medium bowl, toss the fish pieces with the olive oil, chili powder, cumin, garlic powder, salt, and pepper until evenly coated.

3. Arrange the seasoned fish pieces in a single layer on the prepared baking sheet.

4. Bake the fish for 12•15 minutes, or until it flakes easily with a fork.

5. Warm the whole wheat tortillas according to package instructions.

6. To assemble the tacos, place a few pieces of the baked fish in the center of each tortilla. Top with shredded cabbage, diced avocado, red onion, and chopped cilantro.

7. Serve the fish tacos immediately, with lime wedges and salsa or hot sauce on the side, if desired.

Tips:
• Use a variety of white fish fillets, such as cod, tilapia, or halibut, for different flavors.
• Swap the whole wheat tortillas for corn tortillas or lettuce wraps for a low•carb option.
• Add a drizzle of creamy lime or chipotle sauce for extra flavor.
• Encourage teens to customize their tacos with their favorite toppings.
• Serve the baked fish tacos with a side of black beans or a fresh salad for a complete meal.

INGREDIENTS

- 1 pomegranate

23. Pomegranate seeds

INSTRUCTIONS

1. Lay the whole wheat tortillas or wraps out on a clean surface.

2. Spread about 1/4 cup of hummus evenly onto the center of each tortilla.

3. Top the hummus with the shredded carrots, sliced cucumber, baby spinach leaves, diced bell pepper, and diced red onion.

4. Season with a pinch of salt and pepper.

5. Fold the bottom of the wrap up over the filling, then fold in the sides and continue rolling up tightly into a wrap.

6. Cut the wraps in half diagonally to serve.

Tips:
• Use a variety of colorful vegetables like zucchini, tomatoes, or avocado.
• Try different flavors of hummus, like roasted red pepper or garlic herb.
• Add a sprinkle of feta cheese or a drizzle of balsamic glaze for extra flavor.
• Serve the vegetable and hummus wraps with a side of fresh fruit or baked chips for a complete meal.
• Prepare the wraps in advance and refrigerate for a quick and easy lunch or snack.

This vegetable and hummus wrap is a nutritious and satisfying option for teenage boys. The combination of fiber•rich vegetables, protein•packed hummus, and whole grain wrap makes it a well•balanced and flavorful meal.

INGREDIENTS

- 2-3 kiwi fruits

INSTRUCTIONS

1. In a shallow dish, combine the olive oil, garlic powder, oregano, paprika, salt, and pepper. Add the steak and turn to coat both sides evenly with the marinade.

2. Cover the dish and let the steak marinate in the refrigerator for 30 minutes to 1 hour.

3. Preheat your grill or grill pan to medium•high heat.

4. Grill the steak for 4•6 minutes per side, depending on thickness, until it reaches your desired level of doneness. Use a meat thermometer to ensure the steak reaches an internal temperature of 145°F (63°C) for medium•rare, or 160°F (71°C) for medium.

5. Transfer the grilled steak to a cutting board and let it rest for 5•10 minutes before slicing against the grain into thin strips.

Tips:
• For extra flavor, try marinating the steak in a mixture of soy sauce, Worcestershire sauce, and Dijon mustard.
• Experiment with different seasoning blends, like Cajun, Italian, or Southwest•inspired.
• Grill the steak over high heat for a nice char on the outside, then finish cooking over medium heat.
• Serve the grilled steak with roasted potatoes, a fresh salad, or grilled vegetables for a complete meal.
• Slice the steak and use it in wraps, tacos, or over a bed of greens for a quick and easy lunch or dinner.

This grilled lean steak is a delicious and nutritious option for teenage boys. The combination of protein•rich meat, bold seasonings, and a quick cooking method makes it a satisfying and flavorful meal.

INGREDIENTS

- 2 ripe mangoes, peeled, pitted, and diced
- 1 cup diced cucumber
- 1/2 cup diced red onion
- 1/4 cup chopped fresh cilantro
- 2 tbsp fresh lime juice
- 1 tbsp olive oil
- 1/4 tsp salt
- 1/4 tsp black pepper

25. Mango salad

INSTRUCTIONS

1. In a large bowl, whisk together the whole wheat flour, rolled oats, baking powder, and salt.

2. In a separate bowl, whisk together the honey/maple syrup, milk, egg, and melted butter/oil.

3. Pour the wet ingredients into the dry ingredients and stir just until combined (do not overmix).

4. Preheat a waffle iron and lightly grease if needed. Scoop the batter onto the hot waffle iron and cook for 3•5 minutes until golden brown.

5. Serve the waffles warm, topped with the fresh or frozen fruit of your choice. You can also add a drizzle of extra honey or maple syrup if desired.

Enjoy your wholesome and delicious whole grain waffles with nutritious fruit toppings!

INGREDIENTS

- 1 ripe papaya, halved and seeded
- 1 lime, cut into wedges

26. Papaya with lime

1. In a large bowl, mash the black beans with a fork or potato masher until slightly chunky.

2. Add the cooked quinoa, rolled oats, grated carrot, diced onion, minced garlic, chili powder, cumin, smoked paprika, salt, and pepper. Mix well until fully combined.

3. Divide the veggie burger mixture into 4 equal portions and shape them into patties, about 4•5 inches wide and 1/2 inch thick.

4. Heat a large skillet or griddle over medium heat. Cook the veggie burgers for 4•5 minutes per side, or until they are lightly browned and heated through.

5. Toast the whole wheat burger buns while the veggie burgers are cooking.

6. Place the cooked veggie burgers on the toasted buns and top with your desired toppings.

Tips:
• For extra protein, add a tablespoon of nut butter or a sprinkle of shredded cheese to the veggie burger mixture.
• Experiment with different spice blends, like Italian seasoning or Southwest•inspired flavors.
• Make a double batch and freeze the uncooked patties for easy meal prep.
• Serve the veggie burgers with baked sweet potato fries or a fresh salad for a complete meal.
• Encourage teens to get creative with their burger toppings and customizations.

This veggie burger is a nutritious and satisfying option for teenage boys. The combination of fiber•rich beans, whole grains, and nutrient•dense veggies makes it a well•balanced and flavorful meal.

INGREDIENTS

- 1 lb fresh cherries, washed and stems removed

INSTRUCTIONS

1. Preheat oven to 400°F. Season the chicken breasts with the garlic powder, oregano, salt and pepper.

2. Heat the olive oil in a large skillet over medium•high heat. Add the chicken and cook for 3•4 minutes per side until browned.

3. Transfer the skillet to the oven and bake for 15•20 minutes until the chicken is cooked through. Allow to cool slightly, then slice or shred the chicken.

4. In a large salad bowl, combine the chopped romaine, croutons, Parmesan cheese and sliced/shredded chicken.

5. Drizzle the Caesar dressing over the top and toss everything together until well coated.

6. Serve immediately. You can add extra croutons, Parmesan or dressing on the side if desired.

This hearty salad is packed with protein from the chicken, healthy greens, and classic Caesar flavors that teens are sure to love. The combination of textures and flavors makes it a satisfying main dish salad. Enjoy!

INGREDIENTS

- 4-5 ripe plums

1. Preheat oven to 400°F. Line a baking sheet with parchment paper.

2. Set up a breading station with 3 shallow dishes:
• Dish 1: Place the flour
• Dish 2: Place the beaten eggs
• Dish 3: Mix together the panko, Parmesan, garlic powder, oregano, salt and pepper.

3. Working in batches, dip the zucchini fry shapes first in the flour, shaking off any excess. Then dip in the beaten egg, allowing any excess to drip off.

4. Finally, coat the zucchini in the panko•Parmesan mixture, pressing gently to help it adhere.

5. Arrange the breaded zucchini fries in a single layer on the prepared baking sheet.

6. Bake for 18•22 minutes, flipping halfway, until the fries are golden brown and crispy.

7. Serve the baked zucchini fries immediately, while hot and crispy. You can serve them with a side of marinara sauce, ranch dressing or your favorite dipping sauce.

These baked zucchini fries are a healthier alternative to traditional french fries, but still have a crispy, flavorful coating that teens are sure to love. The Parmesan and panko breadcrumbs give them a nice crunch.

INGREDIENTS

- 1 lb fresh grapes, washed

1. Spread 2 tbsp of peanut butter onto each of 2 slices of whole wheat bread.

2. Arrange the sliced banana evenly over the peanut butter on one of the bread slices.

3. Top the banana with the remaining slice of bread to create 2 peanut butter and banana sandwiches.

Tips:
• Use natural, no•sugar•added peanut butter for a healthier option.
• Try swapping the banana for other fresh fruit like apple slices or strawberries.
• Add a drizzle of honey or a sprinkle of cinnamon for extra flavor.
• For a heartier sandwich, add a slice of low•fat cheese or a few pieces of crispy bacon.
• Cut the sandwiches in half diagonally or into quarters for a fun, portable snack.
• Serve the peanut butter and banana sandwiches with a glass of milk or a side of carrot sticks for a complete and balanced meal.

This peanut butter and banana sandwich is a classic and nutritious option for teenage boys. The combination of protein•rich peanut butter, potassium•packed banana, and fiber•filled whole wheat bread makes it a satisfying and energizing snack or meal.

INGREDIENTS

- 6-8 ripe apricots

1. Preheat grill or grill pan to medium•high heat.

2. In a shallow dish, whisk together the olive oil, balsamic vinegar, oregano, garlic powder, salt and pepper. Add the portobello mushroom caps and toss to coat both sides.

3. Grill the mushrooms for 4•5 minutes per side, until tender and slightly charred.

4. Place the grilled portobello caps on the toasted hamburger buns.

5. Top the mushroom burgers with your desired toppings, such as:
• Lettuce, tomato, onion
• Sliced cheese (cheddar, Swiss, provolone)
• Condiments (ketchup, mustard, mayo, etc.)

6. Serve the grilled portobello mushroom burgers immediately while hot.

These meaty, umami•rich portobello mushroom burgers make a satisfying meatless option that teenage boys are sure to enjoy. The balsamic and herb marinade adds great flavor, and the toppings can be customized to their preferences. Serve with baked fries or a fresh salad for a complete meal.

INGREDIENTS

- 4 boneless, skinless chicken breasts
- 2 tbsp olive oil
- 1 tsp salt
- 1 tsp black pepper
- 1 tsp garlic powder
- 1 tsp dried oregano

31. Grilled chicken breast

1. Preheat oven to 400°F. Grease a baking sheet or use a baking dish.

2. In a medium bowl, mix together the feta, spinach, garlic, 1 tsp olive oil, oregano, salt and pepper.

3. Slice each chicken breast horizontally to create a pocket. Stuff each pocket evenly with the spinach•feta mixture.

4. Set up a breading station with 3 shallow dishes:
• Dish 1: Place the flour
• Dish 2: Place the beaten eggs
• Dish 3: Place the panko breadcrumbs

5. Dredge the stuffed chicken breasts first in the flour, shaking off any excess. Then dip in the beaten egg, allowing excess to drip off. Finally, coat in the panko breadcrumbs, pressing gently to adhere.

6. Place the breaded stuffed chicken breasts on the prepared baking sheet or in the baking dish. Drizzle the remaining 2 tsp olive oil over the top.

7. Bake for 25•30 minutes, until the chicken is cooked through and the breading is golden brown.

8. Serve the spinach and feta stuffed chicken breasts hot. Pair with roasted vegetables, rice, or a fresh salad for a complete meal.

This dish is packed with protein, veggies, and bold Mediterranean flavors that teenage boys are sure to love. The crispy breading and creamy feta•spinach filling make it extra satisfying.

INGREDIENTS

- 1 lb ground turkey
- 1/2 cup breadcrumbs
- 1/4 cup grated Parmesan cheese
- 1 egg
- 2 cloves garlic, minced
- 1 tsp dried oregano
- 1/2 tsp salt
- 1/4 tsp black pepper

Instructions

1. Preheat oven to 400°F. Line a baking sheet with parchment paper.

2. In a large bowl, combine all the meatball ingredients and mix well until fully incorporated.

3. Roll the mixture into 1•inch meatballs and place them on the prepared baking sheet.

4. Bake the meatballs for 18•20 minutes, until cooked through.

5. While the meatballs are baking, bring a large pot of salted water to a boil. Cook the whole grain spaghetti according to package instructions until al dente. Drain and set aside.

6. In a large skillet or pot, heat the marinara sauce over medium heat. Add the cooked meatballs and toss to coat.

7. Add the cooked spaghetti to the sauce and meatballs. Toss everything together until well combined.

8. Serve the whole grain spaghetti and turkey meatballs hot, garnished with fresh chopped basil if desired.

This dish provides a nutritious and satisfying meal for teenage boys, with the whole grain pasta, lean turkey meatballs, and flavorful marinara sauce. The combination of flavors and textures is sure to be a hit.

INGREDIENTS

- 1 block (14 oz) firm or extra-firm tofu, cubed
- 2 tbsp vegetable or sesame oil
- 2 cloves garlic, minced
- 1 inch piece fresh ginger, peeled and grated
- 1 red bell pepper, sliced
- 1 cup broccoli florets
- 2 cups sliced mushrooms
- 2 tbsp low-sodium soy sauce
- 1 tbsp rice vinegar
- 1 tsp sesame oil
- Salt and pepper to taste
- Cooked rice or noodles, for serving

INSTRUCTIONS

1. In a large pot or Dutch oven, heat the olive oil over medium heat. Add the onion, carrots, and celery. Cook for 5•7 minutes until softened.

2. Add the garlic, thyme, oregano, paprika, and red pepper flakes (if using). Cook for 1 minute until fragrant.

3. Pour in the broth and diced tomatoes. Bring to a simmer.

4. Add the kidney beans, chickpeas, and chopped kale/spinach. Simmer for 10•15 minutes, until the vegetables are tender.

5. Season with salt and pepper to taste.

6. Serve the vegetable and bean soup hot, with crusty bread or rolls on the side. You can also top with shredded cheese, croutons, or a dollop of sour cream if desired.

This hearty, veggie•packed soup is full of fiber, protein, and nutrients that will keep teenage boys feeling satisfied. The combination of beans, greens, and aromatic spices makes it a nutritious and flavorful meal.

INGREDIENTS

- 1 tbsp olive oil
- 1 onion, diced
- 3 cloves garlic, minced
- 2 carrots, peeled and diced
- 2 celery stalks, diced
- 1 cup dried brown or green lentils, rinsed
- 6 cups low-sodium vegetable or chicken broth
- 1 (14.5 oz) can diced tomatoes
- 1 tsp ground cumin
- 1 tsp dried oregano
- 1/2 tsp smoked paprika
- Salt and pepper to taste
- Chopped parsley or cilantro for garnish (optional)

34. Lentil soup

1. Preheat a large skillet or griddle over medium heat.

2. Lay 4 slices of the whole grain bread on a clean surface. Top each slice with 2 slices of cheddar cheese and a few slices of tomato.

3. Place the remaining 4 slices of bread on top to make 4 sandwiches.

4. Spread the softened butter evenly on the outside of each sandwich.

5. Carefully place the sandwiches in the preheated skillet or griddle. Cook for 3•4 minutes per side, until the bread is golden brown and the cheese is melted.

6. Remove the grilled cheese sandwiches from the heat and let cool for 2•3 minutes before serving.

7. Serve the grilled cheese on whole grain bread with tomato warm, with any desired dipping sauces on the side (such as marinara, ranch, or barbecue sauce).

Tips:
• Use your favorite type of cheddar cheese, or try a blend of cheeses like cheddar and Gruyère.
• Add a sprinkle of dried oregano or Italian seasoning to the tomato slices for extra flavor.
• For a heartier meal, serve the grilled cheese with a side salad or cup of tomato soup.

This classic grilled cheese sandwich gets a nutritious boost from the whole grain bread and fresh tomato slices. Teenage boys are sure to love the gooey, melty cheese and comforting flavors.

INGREDIENTS

- 1 (15 oz) can black beans, rinsed and drained
- 1 cup diced cucumber
- 1 cup diced tomatoes
- 1/2 cup diced red onion
- 1/2 cup diced bell pepper (any color)
- 2 tbsp chopped fresh cilantro
- 2 tbsp lime juice
- 1 tbsp olive oil
- 1 tsp ground cumin
- 1/4 tsp salt
- 1/4 tsp black pepper

INSTRUCTIONS

1. Preheat oven to 400°F. Line a baking sheet with parchment paper.

2. In a food processor, combine the chickpeas, parsley, cilantro, garlic, cumin, coriander, baking soda, and cayenne (if using). Pulse until a coarse paste forms.

3. Transfer the chickpea mixture to a bowl and stir in the flour and olive oil until well combined. Season with salt and pepper.

4. Scoop heaping tablespoons of the falafel mixture and shape into small patties, about 1•inch thick. Place them on the prepared baking sheet.

5. Bake the falafel for 18•22 minutes, flipping halfway, until golden brown and crispy.

6. Serve the baked falafel warm, stuffed into pita bread or naan with chopped tomatoes, cucumbers, red onion, and a drizzle of tahini sauce or tzatziki.

These baked falafel are a healthier alternative to the traditional fried version, but still have a crispy exterior and flavorful interior. Teenage boys will love the Middle Eastern spices and the ability to customize their falafel sandwiches.

INGREDIENTS

- 2 tbsp olive oil
- 1 onion, diced
- 3 cloves garlic, minced
- 1 tbsp grated fresh ginger
- 2 tsp garam masala
- 1 tsp ground cumin
- 1 tsp ground coriander
- 1/2 tsp ground turmeric
- 1/4 tsp cayenne pepper (optional)
- 1 (15 oz) can chickpeas, rinsed and drained
- 1 (14 oz) can diced tomatoes
- 1 cup vegetable or chicken broth
- 1 cup coconut milk
- Salt and pepper to taste
- Chopped cilantro for garnish

1. In a small bowl, mix together the cream cheese, cilantro, garlic powder, salt and pepper until well combined.

2. Lay the turkey slices out flat on a clean surface. Spread a thin layer of the cream cheese mixture evenly over each slice.

3. Place a few slices of avocado in the center of each turkey slice.

4. Carefully roll up the turkey slices around the avocado, securing them with toothpicks if needed.

5. Slice the roll•ups into 2•3.pieces each and arrange on a serving plate.

6. Serve the turkey and avocado roll•ups immediately, or refrigerate until ready to serve.

Tips:
• Use your favorite type of deli turkey, such as smoked, honey roasted, or oven•roasted.
• For extra flavor, you can also add a sprinkle of shredded cheese or a drizzle of balsamic glaze.
• Serve the roll•ups with additional fresh veggies, crackers, or pita chips for dipping.

These turkey and avocado roll•ups make a great snack or light meal for teenage boys. They're packed with protein, healthy fats, and fresh flavors. The creamy avocado and savory turkey are a winning combination.

INGREDIENTS

- 4 (6 oz) salmon fillets, skin-on or skinless
- 1 tbsp lemon juice
- 1 tsp olive oil
- 1/2 tsp salt
- 1/4 tsp black pepper
- Lemon wedges for serving (optional)

37. Steamed salmon

INSTRUCTIONS

1. Heat 1 tbsp of the sesame oil in a large skillet or wok over medium•high heat. Pour in the beaten eggs and cook, stirring occasionally, until scrambled and cooked through. Transfer the eggs to a plate and set aside.

2. In the same skillet, heat the remaining 1 tbsp of sesame oil. Add the frozen mixed vegetables, onion, and garlic. Sauté for 5•7 minutes until the vegetables are tender.

3. Add the chilled cooked brown rice to the skillet. Stir to combine and let the rice heat through, about 2•3 minutes.

4. Pour in the soy sauce, rice vinegar, and ground ginger. Stir to coat the rice and vegetables evenly.

5. Gently fold the cooked scrambled eggs back into the fried rice mixture. Season with salt and pepper to taste.

6. Serve the vegetable fried rice hot, garnished with chopped green onions if desired.

This fried rice dish is packed with veggies, protein from the eggs, and whole grains from the brown rice. The savory Asian•inspired flavors make it a satisfying meal that teenage boys are sure to enjoy. Adjust the seasonings to their preferences.

INGREDIENTS

- 4 (6 oz) cod fillets
- 2 tbsp olive oil
- 1 tsp lemon zest
- 2 tbsp lemon juice
- 2 cloves garlic, minced
- 1 tsp dried parsley
- 1/2 tsp salt
- 1/4 tsp black pepper

INSTRUCTIONS

1. Pat the pork tenderloin dry with paper towels. Place it in a shallow baking dish or resealable plastic bag.

2. In a small bowl, mix together the olive oil, garlic powder, oregano, paprika, salt, and pepper. Rub the seasoning mixture all over the pork tenderloin, making sure to coat it evenly on all sides.

3. Preheat your grill or grill pan to medium•high heat.

4. Place the seasoned pork tenderloin directly on the grill grates. Grill for 12•15 minutes per side, or until the internal temperature reaches 145°F.

5. Transfer the grilled pork tenderloin to a cutting board and let it rest for 5•10 minutes before slicing.

6. Slice the pork tenderloin into 1/2•inch thick medallions and serve immediately.

Serving Suggestions:
• Serve the grilled pork tenderloin with roasted vegetables, mashed potatoes, or a fresh salad.
• Top the pork with a drizzle of barbecue sauce, honey mustard, or chimichurri sauce.
• Use the grilled pork in sandwiches, tacos, or wraps.

This simple grilled pork tenderloin recipe is a great option for teenage boys. The lean protein and bold seasoning make it a satisfying and flavorful main dish. Adjust the cooking time as needed to ensure the pork is cooked through but still juicy.

INGREDIENTS

- 2 (5 oz) cans of tuna, drained
- 1 ripe avocado, diced
- 2 tbsp plain Greek yogurt
- 1 tbsp lemon juice
- 1 tbsp chopped fresh parsley
- 1 tsp Dijon mustard
- 1/4 tsp salt
- 1/4 tsp black pepper

INSTRUCTIONS

1. Preheat grill or grill pan to medium•high heat.

2. In a shallow dish, combine the olive oil, oregano, garlic powder, salt and pepper. Add the chicken breasts and turn to coat both sides.

3. Grill the chicken for 5•7 minutes per side, until cooked through. Let rest for 5 minutes, then slice or chop.

4. In a large salad bowl, combine the chopped romaine, cucumber, tomatoes, red onion, feta, olives and parsley.

5. In a small bowl, whisk together the dressing ingredients.

6. Add the grilled chicken to the salad and drizzle the dressing over the top. Toss everything together until well coated.

7. Serve the Greek salad with grilled chicken immediately.

This colorful and flavorful salad is a great option for teenage boys, with the lean protein from the grilled chicken, healthy fats from the olives and feta, and plenty of fresh veggies. The bold Greek•inspired dressing ties all the flavors together.

INGREDIENTS

- 4 large eggs
- 2 cups water
- 1 tbsp white vinegar
- 1/4 tsp salt

INSTRUCTIONS

1. Preheat oven to 400°F. Line a baking sheet with parchment paper.

2. Pat the tofu sticks dry with paper towels to remove any excess moisture.

3. In a shallow dish, mix together the cornstarch, garlic powder, onion powder, paprika, salt, and pepper.

4. Toss the tofu sticks in the cornstarch mixture, making sure to coat all sides.

5. Arrange the coated tofu sticks in a single layer on the prepared baking sheet. Drizzle the olive oil over the top.

6. Bake for 20•25 minutes, flipping halfway, until the tofu is golden brown and crispy.

7. Remove the baked tofu sticks from the oven and let cool for 5 minutes.

8. Serve the tofu sticks warm, with ranch dressing or another dipping sauce on the side. Garnish with chopped parsley or green onions if desired.

Tips:
• For extra crispy tofu, you can toss the sticks in a bit of cornstarch before coating them.
• Try different seasoning blends like chili powder, cumin, or Italian herbs.
• Serve the baked tofu sticks as a snack or appetizer, or as part of a larger meal.

These baked tofu sticks are a great vegetarian option that teenage boys are sure to enjoy. The crispy exterior and flavorful seasoning make them a tasty and protein•packed alternative to traditional fried snacks.

INGREDIENTS

- 6 large eggs

41. Hard-boiled eggs

INSTRUCTIONS

1. In a large bowl, whisk together the whole wheat flour, rolled oats, baking powder, baking soda, and salt.

2. In a separate bowl, whisk together the honey/maple syrup, milk, egg, and melted butter/oil.

3. Pour the wet ingredients into the dry ingredients and stir just until combined (do not overmix).

4. Fold in the fresh or frozen berries.

5. Heat a lightly oiled griddle or nonstick skillet over medium heat.

6. Scoop the batter onto the hot surface, using about 1/4 cup for each pancake. Cook for 2•3 minutes per side, until golden brown.

7. Serve the whole grain pancakes warm, drizzled with additional honey or maple syrup. Top with a dollop of whipped cream or Greek yogurt if desired.

These hearty, nutrient•dense pancakes are a great way to start the day for teenage boys. The whole grains, protein from the egg, and antioxidants from the berries make this a balanced and satisfying breakfast. Adjust the sweetness to their preferences.

INGREDIENTS

- 1 cup plain, unsweetened Greek yogurt
- 1 cup fresh berries (such as blueberries, raspberries, or sliced strawberries)
- 1/4 cup granola or crushed nuts

1. In a large pot or Dutch oven, heat the olive oil over medium•high heat. Add the beef cubes and brown on all sides, about 5 minutes total. Transfer the beef to a plate.

2. Add the onion, carrots, celery and garlic to the pot. Cook for 5•7 minutes, stirring occasionally, until the vegetables start to soften.

3. Stir in the thyme, rosemary and bay leaf. Cook for 1 minute until fragrant.

4. Pour in the beef broth and diced tomatoes. Bring to a simmer.

5. Add the browned beef back to the pot, along with the diced potatoes. Simmer for 25•30 minutes, until the beef and potatoes are tender.

6. Stir in the frozen peas and cook for 5 more minutes.

7. Season the stew with salt and pepper to taste.

8. Serve the lean beef and vegetable stew hot, with crusty bread or rolls on the side.

This hearty stew is packed with lean protein from the beef, plus plenty of nutrient•dense vegetables. The combination of flavors and textures makes it a satisfying and wholesome meal for teenage boys. Adjust the seasoning to their preferences.

INGREDIENTS

- 1 lb boneless, skinless chicken breasts, sliced into strips
- 2 bell peppers, sliced into strips
- 1 onion, sliced into strips
- 2 tbsp olive oil
- 1 tbsp fajita seasoning
- 1 tsp cumin
- 1/2 tsp chili powder
- Salt and pepper to taste
- 8-10 whole grain tortillas

43. Baked chicken fajitas with whole grain tortillas

1. Make the mango salsa: In a medium bowl, combine the diced mango, red onion, jalapeño, cilantro, lime juice, and 1/4 tsp salt. Stir to mix well and set aside.

2. Prepare the fish: Pat the fish fillets dry and place them in a shallow dish. Drizzle with the olive oil and sprinkle with the chili powder, garlic powder, salt, and pepper. Rub the seasonings all over the fish.

3. Preheat grill or grill pan to medium•high heat.

4. Grill the fish for 3•5 minutes per side, until it flakes easily with a fork and is cooked through.

5. Transfer the grilled fish to plates and top each fillet with a generous spoonful of the mango salsa.

6. Serve the grilled fish with mango salsa immediately, with any extra salsa on the side.

This dish is a great option for teenage boys • the grilled fish provides lean protein, while the fresh mango salsa adds a burst of sweet and tangy flavor. The vibrant colors and flavors make it an appealing and nutritious meal.

INGREDIENTS

- 1 medium spaghetti squash
- 2 tbsp olive oil
- 1 onion, diced
- 3 cloves garlic, minced
- 1 (28 oz) can diced tomatoes
- 2 tbsp tomato paste
- 1 tsp dried oregano
- 1/2 tsp dried basil
- Salt and pepper to taste
- Grated Parmesan cheese (optional)

44. Spaghetti squash with tomato sauce

1. In a large skillet, heat the olive oil over medium heat. Add the sliced bell pepper and mushrooms. Sauté for 5•7 minutes until the vegetables are tender.

2. Stir in the shredded spinach/kale, chili powder, cumin, garlic powder, salt, and pepper. Cook for 2•3 minutes until the greens are wilted.

3. Remove the vegetable mixture from the heat and stir in the shredded grilled chicken.

4. Lay 4 of the whole wheat tortillas on a clean work surface. Divide the chicken and vegetable mixture evenly among the tortillas, spreading it out to the edges.

5. Sprinkle the shredded Mexican cheese over the filling.

6. Top each quesadilla with the remaining 4 tortillas.

7. Heat a large skillet or griddle over medium heat. Cook the quesadillas for 2•3 minutes per side, until the tortillas are golden brown and the cheese is melted.

8. Cut the quesadillas into wedges and serve warm, with your favorite toppings like salsa, guacamole, or sour cream.

These chicken and veggie quesadillas are a great option for teenage boys • they're packed with protein, fiber, and flavor. The combination of grilled chicken, sautéed veggies, and melty cheese makes for a satisfying and delicious meal.

INGREDIENTS

- 1 lb lean pork tenderloin, cut into 1-inch thick slices
- 2 apples, cored and sliced
- 1 onion, sliced
- 2 tbsp olive oil
- 2 tbsp apple cider vinegar
- 1 tsp Dijon mustard
- 1 tsp dried thyme
- Salt and pepper to taste

INSTRUCTIONS

1. Preheat oven to 400°F. Pierce the sweet potatoes several times with a fork.

2. Place the sweet potatoes directly on the oven rack and bake for 45•60 minutes, until very soft when squeezed.

3. Remove the sweet potatoes from the oven and let cool for 5 minutes.

4. Slice each sweet potato in half lengthwise. Scoop out the flesh into a bowl, leaving a thin layer of sweet potato attached to the skin.

5. Mash the sweet potato flesh lightly with a fork. Stir in the drained and rinsed black beans and salsa until well combined.

6. Spoon the sweet potato and black bean mixture back into the potato skins.

7. Top each stuffed sweet potato half with a sprinkle of shredded cheese.

8. Return the stuffed sweet potatoes to the oven and bake for an additional 10•15 minutes, until the cheese is melted.

9. Remove from oven and garnish with chopped fresh cilantro, if desired.

10. Serve the baked sweet potatoes with black beans warm.

This simple yet satisfying dish provides a great balance of complex carbs, protein, and fiber. Teenage boys are sure to enjoy the sweet and savory flavors. Feel free to adjust the toppings to their preferences.

INGREDIENTS

- 8 oz package of tempeh, cut into 1/2-inch thick slices
- 1/2 cup BBQ sauce (use a store-bought or homemade version)
- 1 tbsp olive oil
- 1 tsp smoked paprika
- 1/2 tsp garlic powder
- Salt and pepper to taste

1. Cook the sushi rice according to package instructions. Transfer to a large bowl and stir in the rice vinegar, sugar, and salt. Let cool to room temperature.

2. Place a sheet of nori on the bamboo sushi mat, shiny side down. Spread about 1/4 of the sushi rice evenly over the nori, leaving a 1•inch border at the top.

3. Arrange a few slices of avocado in a line across the center of the rice. Top with a couple tablespoons of the drained tuna.

4. Starting from the bottom, use the sushi mat to tightly roll up the nori around the fillings. Moisten the top edge with water to seal the roll.

5. Repeat with the remaining nori sheets, rice, avocado, and tuna to make 4 sushi rolls total.

6. Use a sharp knife to slice each sushi roll into 6•8 pieces.

7. Serve the tuna and avocado sushi rolls immediately, with soy sauce and wasabi on the side for dipping.

Tips:
• For extra flavor, you can add a drizzle of spicy mayo or sprinkle of toasted sesame seeds on top.
• Substitute canned salmon or grilled chicken for the tuna, if desired.
These tuna and avocado sushi rolls are a nutritious and satisfying option that teenage boys are sure to enjoy. The combination of fresh ingredients and hands•on assembly makes it a fun and interactive meal.

INGREDIENTS

- 1 block (14 oz) extra-firm tofu, cubed
- 2 tbsp sesame oil
- 2 cloves garlic, minced
- 1 inch fresh ginger, grated
- 1 red bell pepper, sliced
- 1 cup broccoli florets
- 1 cup sliced mushrooms
- 1 cup snow peas or snap peas
- 2 tbsp low-sodium soy sauce or tamari
- 1 tbsp rice vinegar
- 1 tsp sesame seeds
- Salt and pepper to taste

47. Vegetable and tofu stir-fry

INSTRUCTIONS

1. In a large pot or Dutch oven, heat the olive oil over medium heat. Add the onion and cook for 5 minutes until translucent.

2. Stir in the garlic, ginger, garam masala, cumin, coriander, turmeric, and cayenne (if using). Cook for 1 minute until fragrant.

3. Add the chickpeas, diced tomatoes, vegetable broth, cauliflower, and sweet potatoes. Bring to a simmer.

4. Reduce heat to medium•low and let the curry simmer for 15•20 minutes, until the vegetables are tender.

5. Stir in the frozen peas and chopped cilantro. Season with salt and pepper to taste.

6. Serve the vegetable and chickpea curry warm, over steamed basmati rice.

Tips:
• For extra protein, you can add cubed cooked chicken or tofu.
• Adjust the amount of cayenne pepper to control the spice level.
• Garnish with additional cilantro, sliced green onions, or a dollop of plain yogurt.

This flavorful curry is packed with nutritious vegetables, protein•rich chickpeas, and aromatic Indian spices. Teenage boys are sure to enjoy the bold flavors and hearty texture of this vegetarian curry dish.

INGREDIENTS

- 1 lb ground turkey breast
- 1 tbsp Dijon mustard
- 1 tsp Worcestershire sauce
- 1 tsp dried oregano
- 1/2 tsp garlic powder
- 1/4 tsp cayenne pepper (optional)
- Salt and pepper to taste
- 8 large lettuce leaves (such as romaine or bibb)
- Toppings: sliced tomatoes, avocado, onion, pickles, etc.

48. Grilled turkey burgers with lettuce wraps

INSTRUCTIONS

1. Preheat oven to 375°F. Cook the lasagna noodles according to package instructions. Drain and set aside.

2. In a large skillet, cook the ground turkey over medium•high heat until browned and crumbled, 5•7 minutes. Drain any excess fat.

3. Add the diced onion and minced garlic to the skillet. Cook for 2•3 minutes until the onion is translucent.

4. Stir in the oregano, basil, and red pepper flakes (if using). Pour in the marinara sauce and simmer for 5 minutes.

5. In a medium bowl, mix together the ricotta cheese, egg, and Parmesan.

6. Spread 1 cup of the meat sauce in the bottom of a 9x13 inch baking dish. Arrange 3 lasagna noodles over the sauce.

7. Spread half of the ricotta cheese mixture over the noodles, then top with half of the thawed and drained spinach.

8. Spread 1 cup of the meat sauce over the spinach, then sprinkle with 1/2 cup of the mozzarella cheese.

9. Repeat the layers of noodles, ricotta, spinach, sauce, and mozzarella. Top with the remaining 3 lasagna noodles and the remaining meat sauce.

10. Cover the dish with aluminum foil and bake for 30 minutes. Remove the foil and bake for an additional 15 minutes, until the cheese is melted and bubbly. Let the lasagna cool for 10•15 minutes before serving.

INGREDIENTS

For the Sweet Potatoes:
- 4 medium sweet potatoes, scrubbed clean
- 1 tbsp olive oil
- Salt and pepper to taste

For the Black Bean Salsa:
- 1 (15 oz) can black beans, rinsed and drained
- 1 cup diced tomatoes
- 1/2 cup diced red onion
- 1 jalapeño, seeded and diced
- 2 tbsp chopped cilantro
- 2 tbsp lime juice
- 1 tsp ground cumin
- Salt and pepper to taste

49. Baked sweet potato with black bean salsa

1. Preheat grill or grill pan to medium•high heat.

2. In a large bowl, toss the zucchini, bell pepper, and eggplant slices with the olive oil, oregano, garlic powder, salt, and pepper.

3. Grill the vegetable slices for 2•3 minutes per side, until tender and lightly charred.

4. Spread a generous layer of hummus on 4 slices of the whole grain bread.

5. Top the hummus with the grilled vegetable slices, dividing them evenly.

6. Add a handful of baby spinach or arugula on top of the vegetables.

7. Place the remaining 4 slices of bread on top to create the sandwiches.

8. Grill the sandwiches for 2•3 minutes per side, until the bread is toasted and the hummus is warmed through.

9. Slice the grilled vegetable and hummus sandwiches in half and serve immediately.

Tips:
• Try using different types of hummus, such as roasted red pepper or garlic herb.
• Add other grilled or roasted veggies like mushrooms, onions, or asparagus.
• For extra protein, you can add sliced grilled chicken or crumbled feta cheese.

This hearty, vegetarian sandwich is packed with nutrient•dense grilled veggies, creamy hummus, and whole grain bread.

INGREDIENTS

- 8 oz whole grain pasta (such as whole wheat or brown rice pasta)
- 1 cup packed fresh basil leaves
- 1/4 cup pine nuts
- 2 cloves garlic
- 1/4 cup grated Parmesan cheese
- 2 tbsp olive oil
- Salt and pepper to taste
- 1 zucchini, sliced into 1/2-inch thick rounds
- 1 red bell pepper, sliced into strips
- 1 yellow squash, sliced into 1/2-inch thick rounds
- 1 tbsp olive oil
- Salt and pepper

INSTRUCTIONS

1. Preheat oven to 400°F. Line a large baking sheet with parchment paper.

2. In a large bowl, toss the sliced chicken, bell peppers, and onion with the olive oil, chili powder, cumin, garlic powder, smoked paprika, and cayenne (if using). Season with salt and pepper.

3. Spread the chicken and vegetable mixture in a single layer on the prepared baking sheet.

4. Bake for 20•25 minutes, stirring halfway, until the chicken is cooked through and the vegetables are tender.

5. Remove the baked chicken fajita mixture from the oven.

6. Warm the whole wheat tortillas according to package instructions.

7. Serve the baked chicken fajitas warm, allowing everyone to assemble their own with the tortillas and desired toppings.

Suggested Toppings:
• Shredded cheddar or Monterey Jack cheese
• Salsa
• Guacamole
• Sour cream
• Chopped cilantro

This baked chicken fajita recipe is a great option for teenage boys • it's easy to make, full of flavor, and customizable to their tastes. The combination of tender chicken, roasted veggies, and warm tortillas makes for a satisfying and nutritious meal.

INGREDIENTS

- 4 mackerel fillets (about 1 lb total)
- 2 tbsp olive oil
- 1 tbsp lemon juice
- 1 tsp Dijon mustard
- 1 tsp dried thyme
- Salt and pepper to taste
- 1 lb Brussels sprouts, trimmed and halved
- 2 tbsp olive oil
- 1 tbsp balsamic vinegar
- 1 clove garlic, minced
- Salt and pepper to taste

51. Grilled mackerel with roasted Brussels sprouts

INSTRUCTIONS

1. Preheat oven to 400°F. Line a large baking sheet with parchment paper.

2. In a medium saucepan, bring the vegetable/chicken broth to a boil. Stir in the whole wheat couscous, cover, and remove from heat. Let stand for 5•7 minutes until the couscous is tender.

3. Meanwhile, on the prepared baking sheet, toss the diced zucchini, bell pepper, broccoli, cauliflower, and red onion with the olive oil, oregano, garlic powder, and red pepper flakes (if using). Season with salt and pepper.

4. Roast the vegetables for 18•22 minutes, stirring halfway, until tender and lightly browned.

5. Fluff the cooked couscous with a fork and transfer to a large serving bowl.

6. Add the roasted vegetables to the couscous and gently mix to combine.

7. Sprinkle the chopped fresh parsley over the top.

8. Serve the whole grain couscous with roasted vegetables warm.

This dish is a great option for teenage boys • it's packed with fiber, vitamins, and minerals from the whole grains and veggies, but still has a delicious flavor profile. The roasted vegetables add a nice depth of flavor and texture.

INGREDIENTS

- 4 boneless, skinless chicken breasts
- 1 cup uncooked quinoa, rinsed
- 2 cups low-sodium chicken or vegetable broth
- 1 cup chopped broccoli florets
- 1 cup chopped bell peppers (any color)
- 1 cup sliced mushrooms
- 2 tbsp olive oil
- 1 tsp dried thyme
- 1 tsp garlic powder
- Salt and pepper to taste

52. Baked chicken breast with quinoa and vegetables

INSTRUCTIONS

1. In a large pot or Dutch oven, heat the olive oil over medium heat. Add the onion and cook for 5 minutes until translucent.

2. Stir in the garlic, ginger, garam masala, cumin, coriander, turmeric, and cayenne (if using). Cook for 1 minute until fragrant.

3. Add the rinsed lentils, diced tomatoes, and vegetable broth. Bring to a simmer.

4. Reduce heat to medium•low and let the curry simmer for 15•20 minutes, until the lentils are tender.

5. Stir in the chopped cauliflower, sweet potatoes, and frozen peas. Continue simmering for 10•15 minutes, until the vegetables are tender.

6. Remove from heat and stir in the chopped cilantro. Season with salt and pepper to taste.

7. Serve the lentil and vegetable curry warm, over steamed basmati rice.

Tips:
• For extra protein, you can add cubed cooked chicken or tofu.
• Adjust the amount of cayenne pepper to control the spice level.
• Garnish with additional cilantro, sliced green onions, or a dollop of plain yogurt.

This hearty, vegetarian curry is packed with fiber, protein, and nutrients from the lentils, vegetables, and aromatic spices. Teenage boys are sure to enjoy the bold flavors and satisfying texture.

INGREDIENTS

- 1 cup dry brown or green lentils, rinsed
- 4 cups low-sodium vegetable broth
- 1 tbsp olive oil
- 1 onion, diced
- 3 cloves garlic, minced
- 1 tbsp grated fresh ginger
- 2 tsp garam masala
- 1 tsp ground cumin
- 1 tsp ground coriander
- 1/2 tsp cayenne pepper (optional)
- 1 (14 oz) can diced tomatoes
- 1 cup chopped cauliflower florets
- 1 cup chopped sweet potato
- 1 cup chopped spinach or kale
- Salt and pepper to taste
- Chopped cilantro for garnish

53. Lentil and vegetable curry

INSTRUCTIONS

1. In a large bowl, combine the ground turkey, breadcrumbs, egg, onion, garlic powder, oregano, salt, and pepper. Mix gently until just combined, being careful not to overmix.

2. Divide the mixture into 4•6 equal portions and shape into patties, about 1/2 inch thick.

3. Preheat grill or grill pan to medium•high heat. Lightly oil the grates.

4. Grill the turkey burgers for 4•5 minutes per side, or until cooked through and no longer pink in the center. An instant•read thermometer should read 165°F.

5. Serve the grilled turkey burgers on buns with your desired toppings.

Tips:
• For extra flavor, you can add in some shredded cheese, diced jalapeños, or other seasonings to the burger mixture.
• Be gentle when forming the patties to prevent them from becoming dense and tough.
• Don't press down on the burgers while cooking, as this can squeeze out the juices.

Enjoy your juicy and flavorful grilled turkey burgers!

INGREDIENTS

- 1 lb lean beef sirloin or flank steak
- 2 tbsp olive oil, divided
- 1 tsp garlic powder
- 1 tsp dried thyme
- Salt and pepper to taste
- 8 oz sliced mushrooms (such as cremini or shiitake)
- 2 cloves garlic, minced
- 2 tbsp balsamic vinegar
- 2 tbsp chopped fresh parsley

1. In a large pot or Dutch oven, heat the olive oil over medium heat. Add the onion and garlic and cook for 2•3 minutes until fragrant.

2. Add the bell pepper and zucchini and cook for 5 minutes, stirring occasionally, until vegetables start to soften.

3. Stir in the black beans, kidney beans, diced tomatoes, chili powder, cumin, oregano, smoked paprika, and cayenne (if using). Season with salt and pepper.

4. Bring the chili to a simmer and let it cook for 15•20 minutes, stirring occasionally, until the flavors have melded and the vegetables are tender.

5. Serve the chili hot, topped with shredded cheddar cheese, sour cream, and chopped cilantro if desired. Enjoy!

This chili is packed with protein from the beans, lots of veggies, and just the right amount of spice to appeal to hungry teenage boys. It's a hearty, satisfying meal.

INGREDIENTS

- 1 lb cod fillets
- 2 tbsp olive oil
- 1 onion, diced
- 3 cloves garlic, minced
- 1 (14 oz) can diced tomatoes
- 1/4 cup pitted kalamata olives, chopped
- 2 tbsp capers, drained
- 1 tsp dried oregano
- Salt and pepper to taste
- Chopped fresh parsley for garnish

1. Preheat your oven to 400°F (200°C).

2. In a small bowl, whisk together the olive oil, lemon juice, lemon zest, garlic, salt, and pepper.

3. Place the cod fillets in a baking dish or on a rimmed baking sheet. Pour the lemon•garlic mixture over the top, making sure to evenly coat the fish.

4. Bake the cod for 12•15 minutes, or until it flakes easily with a fork and is opaque throughout.

5. Remove the baked cod from the oven and sprinkle with the chopped fresh parsley.

6. Serve the baked cod immediately, with the lemon•garlic sauce spooned over the top.

Tips:
• For extra flavor, you can add a few thin lemon slices on top of the cod before baking.
• Adjust the baking time based on the thickness of your cod fillets. Thicker pieces may require a few extra minutes.
• Serve the baked cod with roasted vegetables, rice, or a fresh salad for a complete and healthy meal.

Enjoy your delicious and easy•to•make baked cod with lemon!

INGREDIENTS

- 8 large eggs
- 1/4 cup milk or unsweetened almond milk
- 1/2 tsp salt
- 1/4 tsp black pepper
- 1 tbsp olive oil
- 1 cup diced bell peppers (any color)
- 1 cup sliced mushrooms
- 1 cup chopped spinach or kale
- 1/2 cup diced onion
- 1/2 cup shredded cheddar or feta cheese

56. Vegetable frittata

1. Make the falafel: In a food processor, combine the chickpeas, parsley, garlic, cumin, baking soda, and cayenne (if using). Pulse until a coarse paste forms.

2. Transfer the chickpea mixture to a bowl and stir in the flour and olive oil until well combined.

3. Scoop heaping tablespoons of the falafel mixture and shape into small patties, about 1•inch thick.

4. Heat a large skillet over medium heat with a thin layer of olive oil. Fry the falafel patties for 2•3 minutes per side until golden brown.

5. Drain the fried falafel on a paper towel•lined plate.

6. To assemble the pitas, stuff each pita half with the fried falafel, chopped tomatoes, cucumbers, red onion, and crumbled feta.

7. Drizzle the pitas with tahini sauce or tzatziki, if desired.

8. Serve the whole grain pita sandwiches immediately.

This falafel pita pocket is a great option for teenage boys • it's packed with protein, fiber, and fresh veggies, but still has the satisfying flavors and textures they crave. The whole grain pita provides complex carbs to keep them full.

INGREDIENTS

- 12 oz cremini or button mushrooms, stems removed and finely chopped
- 1 tbsp olive oil
- 1/2 lb ground turkey
- 2 cloves garlic, minced
- 1 cup fresh spinach, chopped
- 2 tbsp grated Parmesan cheese
- 1 tsp dried oregano
- Salt and pepper to taste

57. Turkey and spinach stuffed mushrooms

1. In a large pot or Dutch oven, heat the olive oil over medium•high heat. Add the chicken and cook for 3•4 minutes, until lightly browned.

2. Add the onion, carrots, celery, and garlic to the pot. Sauté for 5 minutes, stirring occasionally, until the vegetables are starting to soften.

3. Pour in the chicken broth and add the diced potatoes, frozen peas, thyme, oregano, salt, and pepper. Bring the soup to a boil.

4. Reduce the heat to medium•low and let the soup simmer for 15•20 minutes, or until the potatoes are tender and the chicken is cooked through.

5. If desired, stir in the cooked egg noodles and let them heat through for 2•3 minutes.

6. Taste the soup and adjust the seasoning as needed.

7. Serve the chicken and vegetable soup hot, garnished with additional fresh herbs or a sprinkle of Parmesan cheese, if desired.

Tips:
• For extra heartiness, you can add diced cooked bacon or shredded rotisserie chicken to the soup.
• Encourage teen boys to help with the preparation, such as chopping the vegetables or measuring the ingredients.
• Serve the soup with crusty bread or a side salad for a complete and satisfying meal.
• This soup can be made in advance and stored in the refrigerator for up to 4 days or frozen for up to 3 months.

INGREDIENTS

For the Falafel:
- 1 (15 oz) can chickpeas, drained and rinsed
- 1/2 cup fresh parsley, chopped
- 1/4 cup fresh cilantro, chopped
- 2 cloves garlic, minced
- 1 tsp ground cumin
- 1/2 tsp ground coriander
- 1/4 tsp cayenne pepper
- 2 tbsp whole wheat flour
- Salt and pepper to taste

For the Salad:
- 5 oz mixed greens
- 1 cup cherry tomatoes, halved
- 1/2 cucumber, sliced
- 1/4 red onion, thinly sliced
- 1/4 cup crumbled feta cheese
- 2 tbsp tahini dressing (or lemon-garlic dressing)

1. In a large bowl, combine the tofu cubes, zucchini, bell pepper, onion, and mushrooms.

2. In a small bowl, whisk together the olive oil, soy sauce, honey, garlic powder, oregano, salt, and black pepper.

3. Pour the marinade over the tofu and vegetables and toss gently to coat everything evenly.

4. Thread the marinated tofu and vegetables onto skewers, alternating the ingredients.

5. Preheat your grill or grill pan to medium•high heat. Lightly oil the grates.

6. Grill the skewers for 10•12 minutes, turning occasionally, until the vegetables are tender and the tofu is lightly charred.

7. Serve the grilled tofu and vegetable skewers hot, with any remaining marinade drizzled over the top.

Tips:
• For extra flavor, you can marinate the skewers for 30 minutes to an hour before grilling.
• If using wooden skewers, be sure to soak them in water for 30 minutes before assembling the skewers to prevent them from burning.
• Encourage teen boys to get involved in the preparation by letting them help assemble the skewers.
• Serve the skewers with a side of rice or quinoa for a complete and satisfying meal.

Enjoy these delicious and nutritious grilled tofu and vegetable skewers!

INGREDIENTS

For the Mango Salsa:
- 1 ripe mango, diced
- 1/2 red onion, finely chopped
- 1 jalapeño, seeded and minced
- 1/4 cup chopped cilantro
- 2 tbsp lime juice
- 1 tsp olive oil
- Salt and pepper to taste

For the Shrimp:
- 1 lb large shrimp, peeled and deveined
- 2 tbsp olive oil
- 1 tsp chili powder
- 1/2 tsp garlic powder
- Salt and pepper to taste

59. Grilled shrimp with mango salsa

1. In a small bowl, whisk together the soy sauce, brown sugar, cornstarch, and red pepper flakes (if using). Set aside.

2. Heat the vegetable oil in a large skillet or wok over high heat. Add the sliced beef and stir•fry for 2•3 minutes, until the beef is no longer pink. Transfer the beef to a plate.

3. Add the broccoli florets to the hot skillet and stir•fry for 2•3 minutes, until the broccoli is crisp•tender.

4. Add the minced garlic and grated ginger to the skillet and stir•fry for 1 minute, until fragrant.

5. Pour the soy sauce mixture into the skillet and bring to a simmer. Cook for 1•2 minutes, until the sauce has thickened slightly.

6. Return the cooked beef to the skillet and toss everything together until the beef is heated through and coated in the sauce.

7. Serve the beef and broccoli stir•fry immediately over the cooked rice.

Tips:
• For extra flavor, you can add a splash of sesame oil to the stir•fry.
• Encourage teen boys to help with the preparation, such as slicing the beef or measuring the ingredients.
• Serve the stir•fry with steamed rice and some fresh fruit or a simple salad for a well•balanced meal.
• This dish can be easily customized by adding other vegetables, such as carrots, snow peas, or mushrooms.

INGREDIENTS

- 4 whole grain tortillas or wraps
- 1 cup hummus (store-bought or homemade)
- 1 cup sliced cucumber
- 1 cup shredded carrots
- 1 cup baby spinach or arugula
- 1/2 cup sliced bell peppers
- 1/4 cup crumbled feta cheese (optional)

60. Whole grain wrap with hummus and vegetables

INSTRUCTIONS

1. Preheat your oven to 375°F (190°C). Line a baking sheet with parchment paper or a silicone baking mat.

2. In three separate shallow dishes, set up your breading station:
   • In the first dish, place the all•purpose flour.
   • In the second dish, place the beaten eggs.
   • In the third dish, mix together the panko breadcrumbs, 1/2 cup of the Parmesan cheese, oregano, garlic powder, salt, and black pepper.

3. Dip the eggplant slices into the flour, then the egg, and finally the breadcrumb mixture, pressing gently to help the breadcrumbs adhere.

4. Arrange the breaded eggplant slices in a single layer on the prepared baking sheet.

5. Bake the eggplant for 20•25 minutes, flipping halfway through, until golden brown and crispy.

6. Remove the baked eggplant from the oven and top each slice with a spoonful of marinara sauce, followed by a sprinkle of the remaining Parmesan cheese and the shredded mozzarella cheese.

7. Return the eggplant to the oven and bake for an additional 10•15 minutes, or until the cheese is melted and bubbly.

8. Serve the baked eggplant parmesan hot, garnished with fresh basil or parsley, if desired.

Tips:
• Encourage teen boys to help with the breading process, as it can be a fun and engaging task.
• Serve the eggplant parmesan with a side of pasta or a fresh salad for a complete and satisfying meal

INGREDIENTS

For the Salmon:
- 4 (6 oz) salmon fillets
- 1 tbsp olive oil
- 1 tsp lemon zest
- Salt and pepper to taste

For the Dill Sauce:
- 1/2 cup plain Greek yogurt
- 2 tbsp chopped fresh dill
- 1 tbsp lemon juice
- 1 tsp Dijon mustard
- 1 clove garlic, minced
- Salt and pepper to taste

61. Baked salmon with dill sauce

INSTRUCTIONS

1. Lay the whole grain wrap or tortilla flat on a clean surface.

2. Layer the sliced turkey down the center of the wrap.

3. Top the turkey with the mixed vegetables of your choice.

4. If desired, spread a thin layer of hummus or low•fat cream cheese over the vegetables.

5. Season with a pinch of salt and pepper.

6. Carefully roll up the wrap, tucking in the sides as you go.

7. Cut the wrap in half diagonally, if desired, and serve.

This wrap provides a good balance of lean protein, complex carbs, fiber, and vitamins/minerals from the vegetables. The whole grain wrap helps keep teens feeling full and satisfied. Pair this with a piece of fruit, yogurt, or a small bag of nuts for a complete, nutritious lunch.

INGREDIENTS

- 2 tbsp olive oil
- 1 onion, diced
- 3 cloves garlic, minced
- 2 carrots, peeled and diced
- 2 celery stalks, diced
- 1 red bell pepper, diced
- 1 (15 oz) can chickpeas, drained and rinsed
- 1 (14 oz) can diced tomatoes
- 2 cups low-sodium vegetable broth
- 1 tsp dried thyme
- 1 tsp paprika
- 1/2 tsp ground cumin
- Salt and pepper to taste
- Chopped parsley for garnish

62. Vegetable and chickpea stew

INSTRUCTIONS

1. Cook the lo mein or udon noodles according to the package instructions. Drain and rinse with cold water. Set aside.

2. In a large skillet or wok, heat 1 tbsp of the sesame oil over medium•high heat. Add the chicken and stir•fry for 5•7 minutes, until cooked through. Transfer the chicken to a plate.

3. Add the remaining 1 tbsp of sesame oil to the skillet. Stir in the garlic and ginger, and cook for 1 minute, until fragrant.

4. Add the mushrooms, cabbage, carrots, and snow peas to the skillet. Stir•fry for 3•5 minutes, until the vegetables are tender•crisp.

5. Return the cooked chicken to the skillet, along with the cooked noodles, soy sauce, and rice vinegar. Toss everything together until well combined and heated through.

6. Serve the vegetable and chicken lo mein hot, garnished with sesame seeds and sliced green onions, if desired.

Tips:
• Encourage teen boys to help with the preparation, such as chopping the vegetables or measuring the ingredients.
• For extra protein, you can add some cooked shrimp or tofu to the lo mein.
• Customize the vegetables based on your teen's preferences, such as adding broccoli, bell peppers, or bean sprouts.
• Serve the lo mein with a side of steamed rice or a fresh salad for a well•balanced meal.

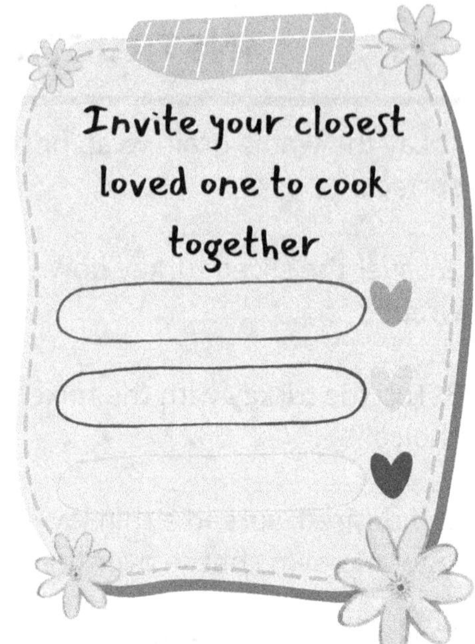

INGREDIENTS

For the Chicken:
- 4 boneless, skinless chicken breasts
- 2 tbsp olive oil
- 1 tsp dried thyme
- 1 tsp garlic powder
- Salt and pepper to taste

For the Roasted Vegetables:
- 2 medium carrots, peeled and cut into 1-inch pieces
- 2 parsnips, peeled and cut into 1-inch pieces
- 1 medium sweet potato, peeled and cut into 1-inch cubes
- 1 red onion, cut into wedges
- 2 tbsp olive oil
- 1 tsp dried rosemary
- Salt and pepper to taste

63. Grilled chicken with roasted root vegetables

INSTRUCTIONS

1. In a large bowl, combine the chopped salmon, panko breadcrumbs, mayonnaise, Dijon mustard, lemon juice, dill, salt, and black pepper. Mix gently until just combined.

2. Divide the salmon mixture into 4 equal portions and shape them into patties, about 1/2 inch thick.

3. Preheat your grill or grill pan to medium•high heat. Lightly oil the grates.

4. Grill the salmon burgers for 4•5 minutes per side, or until they are cooked through and flake easily with a fork.

5. Serve the grilled salmon burgers on the toasted buns, topped with your desired toppings.

Tips:
• For extra flavor, you can add some finely chopped onion or garlic to the salmon mixture.
• Encourage teen boys to get involved in the preparation by letting them help shape the patties.
• Serve the salmon burgers with a side of grilled vegetables or a fresh salad for a well•balanced meal.
• If you prefer a firmer texture, you can chill the salmon mixture in the refrigerator for 30 minutes before forming the patties.

Enjoy these delicious and nutritious grilled salmon burgers!

INGREDIENTS

For the Tofu:
- 1 block (14 oz) extra-firm tofu, pressed and cubed
- 2 tbsp low-sodium soy sauce
- 1 tbsp sesame oil
- 1 tsp cornstarch

For the Stir-Fry:
- 2 tbsp sesame oil
- 3 cloves garlic, minced
- 1 inch fresh ginger, grated
- 1 red bell pepper, sliced
- 1 cup broccoli florets
- 1 cup sliced mushrooms
- 1 cup snow peas or snap peas
- 2 tbsp low-sodium soy sauce
- 1 tbsp rice vinegar
- 1 tsp sesame seeds
- Salt and pepper to taste
- Cooked brown rice, for serving

64. Baked tofu and vegetable stir-fry

Instructions

1. In a medium bowl, mash the black beans with a fork or potato masher. Stir in the olive oil, cumin, chili powder, garlic powder, and salt until well combined.

2. Lay 4 of the tortillas on a flat surface. Spread the seasoned black bean mixture evenly over the tortillas, leaving a 1/2•inch border.

3. Sprinkle the shredded cheese over the black bean mixture, then top with the remaining 4 tortillas.

4. Heat a large skillet or griddle over medium heat. Cook the quesadillas for 2•3 minutes per side, or until the tortillas are golden brown and the cheese is melted.

5. Cut the quesadillas into wedges and serve hot, with salsa, sour cream, and guacamole on the side, if desired.

Tips:
• Encourage teen boys to get involved in the preparation by letting them help mash the beans or assemble the quesadillas.
• For extra flavor, you can add diced jalapeños, sautéed onions, or cooked ground turkey or chicken to the bean mixture.
• Serve the quesadillas with a side of rice and beans or a fresh salad for a more substantial meal.
• Leftovers can be stored in the refrigerator for up to 3 days and reheated in the microwave or on the stovetop.

Enjoy these delicious and easy•to•make bean and cheese quesadillas!

Ingredients

- 1 lb ground turkey
- 1 tbsp olive oil
- 1 onion, diced
- 3 cloves garlic, minced
- 2 bell peppers, diced
- 2 (15 oz) cans kidney beans, drained and rinsed
- 1 (15 oz) can black beans, drained and rinsed
- 1 (28 oz) can diced tomatoes
- 2 tbsp chili powder
- 1 tsp ground cumin
- 1 tsp dried oregano
- 1/2 tsp smoked paprika
- 1/4 tsp cayenne pepper (optional)
- Salt and pepper to taste
- Chopped cilantro for garnish

65. Turkey chili with beans

INSTRUCTIONS

1. Preheat your oven to 375°F (190°C).

2. In a large skillet, cook the ground turkey or beef over medium heat until browned and crumbled, about 5•7 minutes. Drain any excess fat.

3. Add the diced onion and minced garlic to the skillet. Cook for 2•3 minutes, until the onion is translucent.

4. Stir in the cooked rice, diced tomatoes, oregano, basil, salt, and black pepper. Mix well and let the mixture simmer for 5 minutes.

5. Arrange the hollowed•out bell peppers in a baking dish. Stuff each pepper cavity with the ground meat and rice mixture, packing it in tightly.

6. Top each stuffed pepper with a generous amount of shredded mozzarella cheese.

7. Cover the baking dish with foil and bake for 30 minutes.

8. Remove the foil and continue baking for an additional 10•15 minutes, or until the peppers are tender and the cheese is melted and bubbly.

9. Serve the baked stuffed bell peppers hot, garnished with fresh parsley or basil, if desired.

Tips:
• Encourage teen boys to help with the preparation, such as scooping out the pepper seeds or stuffing the peppers.
• For extra flavor, you can add some diced jalapeño or crushed red pepper flakes to the filling.

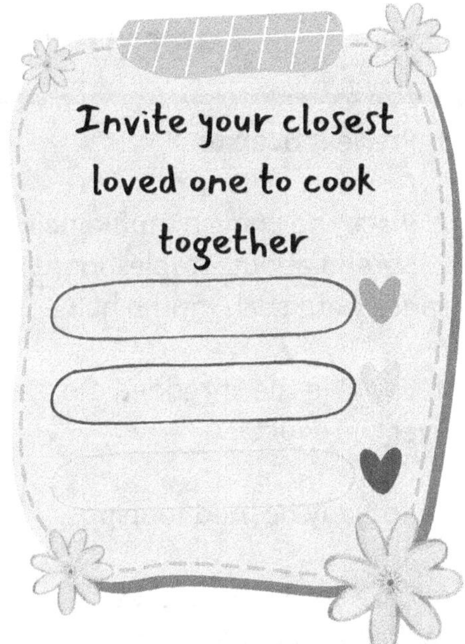

INGREDIENTS

- 8 fresh sardine fillets
- 2 tbsp olive oil
- 3 cloves garlic, minced
- 1 tbsp lemon juice
- 1 tsp lemon zest
- Salt and pepper to taste
- Lemon wedges for serving

66. Grilled sardines with garlic and lemon

INSTRUCTIONS

1. Preheat oven to 400°F.

2. Place the English muffin halves on a baking sheet.
3. Spread about 2 tablespoons of pizza or marinara sauce onto each muffin half.

4. Sprinkle the shredded mozzarella cheese evenly over the sauce.

5. Add any desired toppings.

6. Bake for 8•10 minutes, or until the cheese is melted and bubbly.

7. Let cool for 2•3 minutes before serving.

This recipe is great for teen boys because:
• Whole grain English muffins provide complex carbs and fiber to keep them full.

• The pizza toppings allow for customization to their tastes.

• It's a quick and easy meal that they can make themselves.

• The individual serving size is perfect for a snack or light meal.

• The flavors are familiar and appealing to most teens.

Overall, this whole grain English muffin pizza is a nutritious and delicious option that teen boys are sure to enjoy!

INGREDIENTS

- 1 medium eggplant, sliced into 1/2-inch thick rounds
- 1 cup whole wheat breadcrumbs
- 1/2 cup grated Parmesan cheese
- 1 tsp dried oregano
- 1/2 tsp garlic powder
- 1/4 tsp salt
- 1/4 tsp black pepper
- 1 egg, beaten
- 1 cup marinara sauce
- 1 cup shredded part-skim mozzarella cheese

INSTRUCTIONS

1. In a large skillet or Dutch oven, heat the oil over medium•high heat. Add the chicken and cook for 3•4 minutes until lightly browned. Remove chicken from pan and set aside.

2. Add the onion to the pan and cook for 5 minutes until softened. Add the garlic and ginger and cook for 1 minute until fragrant.

3. Stir in the curry powder, garam masala, cumin, coriander, turmeric and salt. Cook for 1 minute.

4. Add the tomatoes, chicken broth, potatoes and carrots. Bring to a simmer and cook for 10 minutes.

5. Add the cooked chicken, peas and coconut milk. Simmer for 10•15 minutes until chicken is cooked through and vegetables are tender.

6. Garnish with chopped cilantro and serve over basmati rice.

INGREDIENTS

- 1 cup uncooked quinoa, rinsed
- 2 cups low-sodium vegetable or chicken broth
- 1 cup diced cucumber
- 1 cup diced tomatoes
- 1/2 cup diced red onion
- 1/2 cup diced bell pepper (any color)
- 1/2 cup crumbled feta cheese
- 2 tbsp chopped fresh parsley
- 2 tbsp olive oil
- 2 tbsp lemon juice
- 1 tsp Dijon mustard
- 1 tsp honey
- Salt and pepper to taste

68. Quinoa salad with mixed vegetables

1. Preheat your grill or grill pan to medium•high heat.

2. In a large bowl, toss the zucchini, bell pepper, and eggplant slices with the olive oil, Italian seasoning, salt, and black pepper.

3. Grill the vegetables for 2•3 minutes per side, or until they are tender and have grill marks.

4. Remove the grilled vegetables from the heat and let them cool slightly.

5. Spread the pesto (if using) on one side of each slice of bread or panini roll.

6. Layer the grilled vegetables and mozzarella cheese slices on the pesto•coated bread.

7. Place the sandwiches on a hot grill or panini press and cook for 3•5 minutes per side, or until the bread is toasted and the cheese is melted.

8. Remove the grilled vegetable and mozzarella panini from the heat and serve immediately.

Tips:
• Encourage teen boys to help with the grilling and assembly of the panini.
• For a heartier option, you can add some grilled chicken or prosciutto to the panini.
• Serve the panini with a side of fresh fruit or a simple salad for a well•balanced meal.
• If you don't have a grill or panini press, you can toast the sandwiches in a skillet or griddle pan.

Enjoy these delicious and satisfying grilled vegetable and mozzarella panini!

INGREDIENTS

For the Pork Chops:
- 4 lean boneless pork chops (about 1 lb total)
- 1 tbsp olive oil
- 1 tsp garlic powder
- 1 tsp dried thyme
- Salt and pepper to taste

For the Applesauce:
- 3 medium apples, peeled, cored and diced
- 2 tbsp water
- 1 tbsp honey
- 1/2 tsp ground cinnamon

69. Grilled lean pork chops with applesauce

INSTRUCTIONS

1. In a large skillet or wok, heat the vegetable oil over medium•high heat. Add the ground turkey and cook, breaking it up with a wooden spoon, until browned and cooked through, about 5•7 minutes. Transfer the turkey to a plate and set aside.

2. Add the onion to the skillet and cook for 2•3 minutes until softened. Add the garlic and ginger and cook for 1 minute until fragrant.

3. Add the bell pepper, broccoli, mushrooms and snow peas to the skillet. Stir•fry for 4•5 minutes until the vegetables are tender•crisp.

4. Return the cooked turkey to the skillet. Add the soy sauce, rice vinegar, sesame oil and red pepper flakes (if using). Toss everything together and cook for 2•3 minutes until heated through.

5. Season with salt and pepper to taste.

6. Serve the turkey and vegetable stir•fry over steamed rice.

INGREDIENTS

- 4 cod fillets (about 1 lb total)
- 3 cloves garlic, minced
- 2 tbsp fresh parsley, chopped
- 1 tbsp fresh thyme, chopped
- 1 tbsp fresh rosemary, chopped
- 2 tbsp olive oil
- Salt and pepper to taste

70. Baked cod with garlic and herbs

1. Preheat your oven to 375°F (190°C). Line two large baking sheets with parchment paper.

2. In a large bowl, toss the sliced zucchini, carrots, and sweet potato with the olive oil, garlic powder, onion powder, paprika, salt, and pepper until the veggies are evenly coated.

3. Arrange the veggie slices in a single layer on the prepared baking sheets, making sure they are not overlapping.

4. Bake for 18•22 minutes, flipping the veggie slices halfway through, until they are crispy and lightly browned.

5. Remove the baked veggie chips from the oven and let them cool on the baking sheets for 5 minutes before serving.

These baked veggie chips are a healthier alternative to traditional potato chips, but they still have a satisfying crunch and flavor that teenage boys will love. The combination of zucchini, carrots, and sweet potato provides a variety of nutrients and colors.

Serve these veggie chips as a snack or side dish. They're great for packing in lunchboxes or enjoying as a movie night treat. Encourage your teenage boys to get creative and try different seasoning blends to find their favorite flavor.

INGREDIENTS

- 1 tablespoon olive oil
- 1 onion, diced
- 3 cloves garlic, minced
- 2 carrots, peeled and diced
- 2 celery stalks, diced
- 1 cup green or brown lentils, rinsed
- 6 cups vegetable or chicken broth
- 1 (14.5 oz) can diced tomatoes
- 2 bay leaves
- 1 teaspoon dried thyme
- 1 teaspoon dried oregano
- Salt and pepper to taste
- Chopped parsley for garnish (optional)

71. Vegetable and lentil soup

1. Cook the pasta according to package instructions. Drain and rinse with cold water to cool.

2. In a large bowl, combine the cooked and cooled pasta, grilled chicken, cherry tomatoes, cucumber, red onion, feta cheese, and fresh basil.

3. In a small bowl, whisk together the olive oil, red wine vinegar, Dijon mustard, and dried oregano. Season with salt and pepper to taste.

4. Pour the dressing over the pasta salad and toss gently to coat everything evenly.

5. Refrigerate the pasta salad for at least 30 minutes to allow the flavors to meld.

6. Serve chilled or at room temperature.

This pasta salad is a great option for teenage boys because it's packed with protein from the chicken, fiber from the whole grain pasta, and a variety of fresh vegetables. The tangy dressing and feta cheese add lots of flavor. It's a perfect lunch or light dinner that's easy to make and satisfying to eat.

INGREDIENTS

- 4 boneless, skinless chicken breasts
- 1 romaine lettuce heart, chopped
- 1/2 cup croutons
- 1/4 cup grated Parmesan cheese
- 2 tbsp lemon juice
- 2 tbsp olive oil
- 1 tbsp low-fat mayonnaise
- 1 tsp Dijon mustard
- 1 garlic clove, minced
- Salt and pepper to taste

72. Grilled chicken Caesar salad (light dressing)

INSTRUCTIONS

1. In a large pot or Dutch oven, heat the olive oil over medium heat. Add the onion and sauté for 5 minutes until translucent.

2. Add the garlic and sauté for 1 minute until fragrant.

3. Stir in the lentils, broth, diced tomatoes, cumin, oregano, and smoked paprika. Season with salt and pepper to taste.

4. Bring the soup to a boil, then reduce heat and let it simmer for 20•25 minutes, or until the lentils are tender.

5. Stir in the chopped spinach and let it wilt down, about 2•3 minutes.

6. Serve the lentil and spinach soup hot, garnished with grated Parmesan cheese if desired.

This soup is packed with protein from the lentils, and the spinach provides a boost of vitamins and minerals. The smoky, savory flavors will appeal to teenage boys' tastes. Serve it with some crusty bread or a side salad for a complete and satisfying meal.

INGREDIENTS

- 4 medium sweet potatoes
- 1 cup plain Greek yogurt
- 2 tbsp honey
- 1 tsp ground cinnamon
- 1/4 tsp ground nutmeg
- Pinch of salt

73. Baked sweet potato with Greek yogurt topping

INSTRUCTIONS

1. In a large bowl, combine the chicken cubes, pineapple cubes, olive oil, brown sugar, soy sauce, garlic powder, ground ginger, salt, and black pepper. Toss to coat everything evenly.

2. Thread the chicken and pineapple cubes onto the skewers, alternating between the two.

3. Preheat your grill to medium·high heat.

4. Grill the skewers for 12·15 minutes, turning occasionally, until the chicken is cooked through and the pineapple is lightly charred.

5. Serve the grilled chicken and pineapple skewers immediately.

These skewers are a great option for teenage boys because they combine the savory flavors of grilled chicken with the sweet and tangy pineapple. The brown sugar and soy sauce marinade adds a delicious caramelized glaze to the skewers.

Serve the skewers with some rice or a fresh salad for a complete and satisfying meal. You can also offer some dipping sauces like teriyaki or sweet chili sauce on the side.

Grilling the skewers is a fun and interactive way to get teenage boys involved in the cooking process. Encourage them to help assemble the skewers and take turns flipping them on the grill.

INGREDIENTS

- 1 lb ground turkey
- 1 red bell pepper, cut into 1-inch pieces
- 1 zucchini, cut into 1-inch pieces
- 1 red onion, cut into 1-inch pieces
- 8 oz mushrooms, halved
- 2 tbsp olive oil
- 1 tsp dried oregano
- 1 tsp garlic powder
- Salt and pepper to taste

Marinade:
- 2 tbsp lemon juice
- 1 tbsp Dijon mustard
- 1 tbsp honey
- 1 garlic clove, minced
- 1 tsp dried thyme
- 1/4 tsp cayenne pepper

1. Soak the rice noodles in hot water for 15•20 minutes until softened. Drain and set aside.

2. In a large wok or skillet, heat the vegetable oil over medium•high heat. Add the cubed tofu and cook for 3•4 minutes, turning occasionally, until lightly browned. Remove the tofu from the wok and set aside.

3. In the same wok, add the minced garlic and stir•fry for 1 minute until fragrant.

4. Add the carrots, bean sprouts, and broccoli to the wok. Stir•fry for 2•3 minutes until the vegetables are slightly softened.

5. Push the vegetables to the side of the wok and pour the beaten eggs into the center. Scramble the eggs for 1•2 minutes until cooked through.

6. Add the cooked rice noodles, tofu, fish sauce, lime juice, brown sugar, and chili•garlic sauce to the wok. Toss everything together until well combined and heated through.

7. Remove the pad thai from the heat and garnish with chopped roasted peanuts and fresh cilantro.

Serve the vegetable and tofu pad thai immediately, while it's hot and fresh. The combination of flavors and textures will appeal to teenage boys, and the protein•rich tofu and vegetables make it a nutritious meal.

You can adjust the spice level by adding more or less chili•garlic sauce to suit their preferences. Encourage them to customize their pad thai with additional toppings like crushed peanuts, lime wedges, or hot sauce.

INGREDIENTS

- 1 block (14 oz) extra-firm tofu, cut into 4 thick "steaks"
- 2 tbsp vegetable oil
- 1/4 cup low-sodium soy sauce
- 2 tbsp brown sugar
- 2 tbsp rice vinegar
- 1 tbsp sesame oil
- 2 garlic cloves, minced
- 1 tsp grated fresh ginger
- 1/4 tsp red pepper flakes (optional)
- 2 tsp sesame seeds (for garnish)
- Chopped green onions (for garnish)

75. Grilled tofu steaks with teriyaki sauce

1. Preheat your oven to 375°F (190°C).

2. In a large bowl, combine the ground turkey, breadcrumbs, milk, egg, onion, garlic, oregano, basil, salt, and pepper. Mix well until all the ingredients are evenly distributed.

3. Transfer the turkey mixture to a 9x5 inch loaf pan and shape it into a loaf.

4. In a small bowl, mix together the ketchup, brown sugar, and Worcestershire sauce. Spread this mixture evenly over the top of the meatloaf.

5. Bake the meatloaf in the preheated oven for 55•60 minutes, or until the internal temperature reaches 165°F (75°C).

6. Let the meatloaf rest for 5•10 minutes before slicing and serving.

This turkey meatloaf is sure to be a hit with teenage boys! It's hearty, flavorful, and easy to make. Serve it with some mashed potatoes, roasted vegetables, or a fresh salad for a complete and satisfying meal. Enjoy!

INGREDIENTS

- 2 medium zucchini, grated (about 2 cups)
- 1/2 cup all-purpose flour
- 1/4 cup grated Parmesan cheese
- 2 eggs, lightly beaten
- 2 tbsp chopped fresh parsley
- 1 garlic clove, minced
- 1/2 tsp baking powder
- 1/4 tsp salt
- 1/4 tsp black pepper

For the Tuna Salad:
1. In a medium bowl, combine the drained tuna, mayonnaise, Dijon mustard, celery, red onion, parsley, and lemon juice. Mix well until everything is evenly distributed.
2. Season with salt and pepper to taste. Cover and refrigerate until ready to serve.

For the Crackers:
1. Preheat your oven to 400°F (200°C). Line a baking sheet with parchment paper.
2. In a food processor, pulse the whole wheat flour, rolled oats, and salt until the oats are finely ground. Add the cold butter and pulse until the mixture resembles coarse crumbs.
3. Add the cold water 1 tbsp at a time, pulsing after each addition, until the dough just begins to come together.
4. Turn the dough out onto a lightly floured surface and knead briefly until it forms a smooth ball.
5. Roll the dough out to 1/8•inch thickness. Use a cookie cutter or knife to cut the dough into desired cracker shapes.
6. Transfer the crackers to the prepared baking sheet, spacing them about 1 inch apart.
7. Bake for 12•15 minutes, or until the crackers are lightly golden and crisp.
8. Allow the crackers to cool completely on the baking sheet before serving.

To Serve:
Top the whole grain crackers with a spoonful of the tuna salad mixture. Enjoy this healthy and satisfying snack or light meal!

INGREDIENTS

- 8 oz whole grain pasta (such as spaghetti or linguine)
- 2 tbsp olive oil
- 3 garlic cloves, minced
- 1/2 cup dry white wine
- 1 (6.5 oz) can chopped clams, with juice
- 1 (14.5 oz) can diced tomatoes
- 1/4 cup chopped fresh parsley
- 1/4 tsp red pepper flakes (optional)
- Salt and black pepper to taste

1. Preheat your oven to 400°F (200°C).

2. In a large skillet, heat the olive oil over medium•high heat. Add the cubed chicken and cook for 5•7 minutes, until lightly browned. Remove the chicken from the skillet and set aside.

3. In the same skillet, add the onion, carrots, celery, and mushrooms. Sauté for 5•7 minutes, until the vegetables are tender.

4. Add the minced garlic and cook for 1 minute, until fragrant.

5. Sprinkle the flour over the vegetables and stir to coat. Cook for 2 minutes, then gradually whisk in the chicken broth and milk. Bring the mixture to a simmer and cook for 5 minutes, or until thickened.

6. Stir the cooked chicken, thyme, parsley, salt, and pepper into the vegetable mixture.

7. Transfer the chicken and vegetable filling to a 9•inch pie dish.

8. Unfold the thawed puff pastry sheet and place it over the filling, pressing the edges to seal. Cut a few slits in the top of the pastry to allow steam to escape.

9. Bake the pot pie for 25•30 minutes, or until the pastry is golden brown and flaky. Let the pot pie cool for 5•10 minutes before serving.

This chicken and vegetable pot pie is sure to be a hit with teenage boys. The flaky puff pastry crust and hearty filling will satisfy their appetites, while the combination of chicken, vegetables, and savory seasonings provides a delicious and balanced meal.

INGREDIENTS

- 4 trout fillets (about 1 lb total)
- 2 tbsp olive oil
- 2 tbsp fresh lemon juice
- 2 tbsp chopped fresh dill
- 1 tsp grated lemon zest
- 1/2 tsp salt
- 1/4 tsp black pepper

1. Cook the quinoa: In a medium saucepan, combine the quinoa and broth. Bring to a boil, then reduce heat to low, cover and simmer for 15•20 minutes until quinoa is tender. Fluff with a fork.

2. Grill the vegetables: Preheat grill or grill pan to medium•high heat. Brush the zucchini, bell pepper, squash and onion slices with olive oil and season with salt and pepper. Grill for 2•3 minutes per side until charred and tender.

3. Assemble the bowls: Divide the cooked quinoa among 4 bowls. Top each with grilled vegetables, spinach/arugula, feta cheese (if using) and pumpkin seeds (if using).

4. Serve immediately and enjoy! The grilled vegetables and quinoa make a nutritious and flavorful vegetarian meal.

INGREDIENTS

- 8 chicken drumsticks
- 2 tbsp olive oil
- 1 tsp paprika
- 1 tsp garlic powder
- 1 tsp dried thyme
- 1/2 tsp salt
- 1/4 tsp black pepper
- 1 lb carrots, peeled and cut into 1-inch pieces
- 2 tbsp honey

79. Baked chicken drumsticks with roasted carrots

1. In a large bowl, combine the beef cubes, bell pepper pieces, onion, mushrooms, and zucchini rounds.

2. In a small bowl, whisk together the olive oil, Worcestershire sauce, soy sauce, garlic powder, oregano, salt, and black pepper.

3. Pour the marinade over the beef and vegetables and toss to coat everything evenly. Cover and refrigerate for at least 30 minutes, or up to 2 hours.

4. Preheat your grill to medium•high heat.

5. Thread the marinated beef and vegetables onto the skewers, alternating the ingredients.

6. Grill the kabobs for 12•15 minutes, turning occasionally, until the beef is cooked through and the vegetables are tender.

7. Serve the beef and vegetable kabobs immediately, with any remaining marinade drizzled over the top.

These kabobs are a great option for teenage boys because they combine juicy, flavorful beef with a variety of fresh vegetables. The Worcestershire and soy sauce marinade adds a delicious savory•sweet taste.

Grilling the kabobs is a fun and interactive way to get teenage boys involved in the cooking process. Encourage them to help assemble the skewers and take turns flipping them on the grill.

Serve the kabobs with some rice or a fresh salad for a complete and satisfying meal. You can also offer some dipping sauces like teriyaki or barbecue sauce on the side.

INGREDIENTS

- 1 cup cooked brown rice
- 1 (15 oz) can black beans, rinsed and drained
- 1 cup diced bell peppers (mix of red, yellow, and/or orange)
- 1 cup diced zucchini
- 1/2 cup diced red onion
- 1 cup corn kernels (fresh, frozen, or canned)
- 2 tbsp chopped fresh cilantro
- 1 avocado, diced
- 2 tbsp lime juice
- 1 tsp ground cumin
- 1/2 tsp chili powder
- Salt and pepper to taste

Toppings (optional):
- Shredded cheese
- Salsa
- Greek yogurt or sour cream
- Sliced jalapeños

80. Vegetable and bean burrito bowl

1. Preheat your oven to 200°F (95°C). Line 2•3 baking sheets with parchment paper.

2. Wash and core the apples. Slice them into thin, even slices about 1/8 inch thick. You can use a mandoline slicer or a sharp knife.

3. Arrange the apple slices in a single layer on the prepared baking sheets. Make sure they are not overlapping.

4. Brush the apple slices lightly with lemon juice. This will help prevent browning.

5. Sprinkle the apple slices evenly with the ground cinnamon and a pinch of salt, if using.

6. Bake for 2•3 hours, flipping the slices halfway through, until the apples are dried and crispy. The baking time may vary depending on the thickness of the slices and your oven.

7. Once the chips are done, let them cool completely on the baking sheets. They will continue to crisp up as they cool.

8. Store the baked apple chips in an airtight container at room temperature for up to 1 week.

These baked apple chips make a great healthy, crunchy snack for active teen boys. They're packed with fiber, vitamins, and natural sweetness. Enjoy!

INGREDIENTS

For the Chimichurri Sauce:
- 1 cup fresh parsley, finely chopped
- 3 garlic cloves, minced
- 1/4 cup olive oil
- 2 tbsp red wine vinegar
- 1 tbsp fresh oregano, chopped
- 1 tsp red pepper flakes
- 1/2 tsp salt
- 1/4 tsp black pepper

For the Beef:
- 1 lb lean beef tenderloin or flank steak
- 1 tbsp olive oil
- Salt and pepper to taste

81. Grilled lean beef with chimichurri sauce

1. Heat the olive oil in a non•stick skillet over medium heat. Add the diced bell pepper and onion. Sauté for 3•4 minutes until softened.

2. Add the scrambled eggs to the skillet and cook, stirring occasionally, until the eggs are fully cooked, about 2•3 minutes.

3. Remove the egg and veggie mixture from the heat and stir in the chopped spinach/kale. Season with salt and pepper.

4. Lay the whole grain tortillas or wraps on a flat surface. Divide the egg and veggie mixture evenly between the two wraps.

5. Sprinkle the shredded cheese over the top of the egg and veggie mixture.

6. Fold the bottom of the wrap up over the filling, then fold in the sides and continue rolling up tightly to create a wrap.

7. You can serve the wraps immediately, or wrap them in foil or parchment paper to enjoy on•the•go.

This wrap is packed with protein from the eggs, fiber and nutrients from the veggies, and whole grains from the tortilla. It's a balanced and satisfying meal that teen boys are sure to enjoy.

INGREDIENTS

For the Falafel:
- 1 (15 oz) can chickpeas, rinsed and drained
- 1/2 cup fresh parsley, chopped
- 1/4 cup fresh cilantro, chopped
- 2 garlic cloves, minced
- 1 tsp ground cumin
- 1 tsp ground coriander
- 1/2 tsp baking soda
- 1/4 tsp cayenne pepper
- 2 tbsp whole wheat flour
- Salt and pepper to taste

For the Tzatziki Sauce:
- 1 cup plain Greek yogurt
- 1 cucumber, peeled, seeded, and grated
- 1 garlic clove, minced
- 1 tbsp fresh lemon juice
- 1 tbsp chopped fresh dill
- Salt and pepper to taste

82. Baked falafel balls with tzatziki

INSTRUCTIONS

1. Heat the sesame oil in a large skillet or wok over high heat. Add the shrimp and cook for 2•3 minutes until they start to turn pink. Remove the shrimp from the pan and set aside.

2. Add the garlic and ginger to the pan and cook for 1 minute, stirring constantly, until fragrant.

3. Add the bell pepper, broccoli, snap peas, and mushrooms to the pan. Stir•fry for 4•5 minutes until the vegetables are tender•crisp.

4. Return the cooked shrimp to the pan. Add the soy sauce and rice vinegar. Toss everything together and cook for 2 more minutes.

5. Remove from heat and garnish with sliced green onions and sesame seeds (if using).

6. Serve immediately over steamed rice or noodles.

This stir•fry is packed with lean protein from the shrimp, fiber and vitamins from the veggies, and tons of flavor. It's a quick, easy, and nutritious meal that teen boys are sure to love.

INGREDIENTS

- 1 cup dry brown or green lentils, rinsed
- 4 cups low-sodium vegetable broth
- 1 tbsp olive oil
- 1 onion, diced
- 3 garlic cloves, minced
- 2 carrots, peeled and diced
- 2 celery stalks, diced
- 1 red bell pepper, diced
- 1 zucchini, diced
- 1 (15 oz) can diced tomatoes
- 2 tsp dried thyme
- 1 tsp dried oregano
- 1/2 tsp smoked paprika
- Salt and black pepper to taste
- 1/2 cup shredded cheddar or mozzarella cheese (optional)

INSTRUCTIONS

1. Preheat your grill to medium•high heat.

2. In a small bowl, mix together the olive oil, chili powder, cumin, garlic powder, and salt. Brush this seasoning mixture evenly over the fish fillets.

3. Grill the fish for 4•5 minutes per side, or until it flakes easily with a fork.

4. While the fish is grilling, prepare the slaw. In a medium bowl, combine the shredded cabbage, carrots, cilantro, lime juice, olive oil, honey, and salt. Toss to coat everything evenly.

5. Once the fish is cooked, flake it into bite•sized pieces.

6. Warm the tortillas according to package instructions.

7. To assemble the tacos, place some of the grilled fish into each tortilla, then top with the slaw.

8. Serve the fish tacos immediately, with any additional toppings like diced avocado, salsa, or hot sauce on the side.

These grilled fish tacos are a great option for teenage boys because they're packed with flavor, but still relatively healthy. The slaw adds a refreshing crunch and the fish is tender and flaky.

Encourage your teenage boys to get creative with their taco toppings and customize them to their liking. Grilling the fish is also a fun, interactive way to get them involved in the cooking process.

INGREDIENTS

- 1 lb tuna steaks
- 2 tbsp olive oil, plus more for drizzling
- 1 tsp Dijon mustard
- 1 tbsp lemon juice
- 1 tsp dried oregano
- Salt and pepper to taste
- 4 cups mixed greens
- 1 cup cherry tomatoes, halved
- 1 cup cooked green beans, cut into 1-inch pieces
- 1/2 cup Kalamata olives, pitted and halved
- 2 hard-boiled eggs, quartered
- 2 tbsp capers
- 2 tbsp red wine vinegar

84. Grilled tuna nicoise salad

INSTRUCTIONS

1. Preheat oven to 375°F. Cut the tops off the bell peppers and remove the seeds and membranes. Place the peppers in a baking dish.

2. In a large skillet, cook the ground turkey over medium heat until browned and cooked through, 5•7 minutes. Drain any excess fat.

3. Add the onion, zucchini, tomatoes, garlic, oregano, basil, salt and pepper to the skillet. Cook for 5 minutes, stirring occasionally, until the vegetables are tender.

4. Remove the skillet from heat and stir in the cooked brown rice.

5. Stuff the hollowed bell peppers evenly with the turkey and vegetable mixture. Top each stuffed pepper with shredded mozzarella cheese.

6. Cover the baking dish with foil and bake for 25•30 minutes, until the peppers are tender.

7. Remove the foil and bake for an additional 5 minutes to melt and brown the cheese.

8. Serve the stuffed peppers warm. Enjoy!

These turkey and veggie stuffed peppers are a nutritious and satisfying meal for active teen boys. The lean protein, whole grains, and vegetables make it a balanced dish.

INGREDIENTS

For the Meatloaf:
- 1 lb ground turkey
- 1 cup whole wheat breadcrumbs
- 1/2 cup finely chopped onion
- 2 garlic cloves, minced
- 1 egg
- 2 tbsp tomato paste
- 1 tsp dried oregano
- 1/2 tsp salt
- 1/4 tsp black pepper

For the Cauliflower Mash:
- 1 head of cauliflower, cut into florets
- 1/4 cup unsweetened almond milk
- 2 tbsp grated Parmesan cheese
- 1 tbsp olive oil
- 1/2 tsp garlic powder
- Salt and pepper to taste

85. Baked turkey meatloaf with cauliflower mash

INSTRUCTIONS

1. Preheat your oven to 400°F (200°C). Line a large baking sheet with parchment paper.

2. In a large bowl, toss the sweet potato wedges with the olive oil, paprika, garlic powder, salt, and pepper until the wedges are evenly coated.

3. Arrange the seasoned sweet potato wedges in a single layer on the prepared baking sheet, making sure they are not overlapping.

4. Bake for 20•25 minutes, flipping the wedges halfway through, until they are tender and lightly browned on the edges.

5. Remove the baked sweet potato wedges from the oven and let them cool for 5 minutes before serving.

Tips:
• For extra crispiness, you can broil the wedges for 2•3 minutes at the end.
• Try different seasoning blends like chili powder, cumin, or cajun spice.
• Serve the baked sweet potato wedges as a side dish or enjoy them as a healthy snack.

These baked sweet potato wedges are a nutritious and delicious option for active teen boys. They're packed with vitamins, minerals, and complex carbohydrates to provide sustained energy. The crispy exterior and soft interior make them irresistible!

INGREDIENTS

- 1 block (14 oz) extra-firm tofu, cubed
- 2 tbsp coconut oil
- 1 onion, diced
- 3 garlic cloves, minced
- 1 tbsp grated fresh ginger
- 2 tsp curry powder
- 1 tsp ground cumin
- 1/2 tsp ground turmeric
- 1/4 tsp cayenne pepper (optional)
- 1 red bell pepper, sliced
- 1 cup sliced mushrooms
- 1 cup chopped cauliflower florets
- 1 cup chopped broccoli florets
- 1 (13.5 oz) can coconut milk
- 1 cup low-sodium vegetable broth
- 2 tbsp tomato paste
- 1 tsp grated lime zest
- 2 tbsp fresh lime juice
- Salt and black pepper to taste
- Chopped cilantro for garnish

86. Vegetable and tofu curry

INSTRUCTIONS

1. Toast the whole grain bread until lightly golden brown.

2. In a small bowl, mash the avocado with a fork until it reaches your desired consistency. Season with a pinch of salt and pepper.

3. Cook the eggs in a skillet with the olive or avocado oil over medium heat, until they reach your preferred doneness.

4. Spread the mashed avocado evenly over the toasted whole grain bread slices.

5. Top the avocado toast with the cooked eggs.

6. Add any additional desired toppings like sliced tomatoes, red onion, fresh herbs, or a drizzle of hot sauce.

7. Serve the whole grain toast with avocado and egg immediately.

This nutrient•dense breakfast or snack provides a great balance of healthy fats from the avocado, protein from the eggs, and complex carbs from the whole grain bread. It's a satisfying and energizing meal that teen boys are sure to enjoy.

The healthy fats, fiber, and nutrients in this dish will help keep teen boys feeling full and fueled throughout the day. It's a simple yet delicious way to start the day or refuel after sports or activities.

INGREDIENTS

For the Ratatouille:
- 1 medium eggplant, diced
- 1 zucchini, diced
- 1 yellow squash, diced
- 1 red bell pepper, diced
- 1 onion, diced
- 3 garlic cloves, minced
- 2 tbsp olive oil
- 1 (14.5 oz) can diced tomatoes
- 2 tbsp chopped fresh basil
- 1 tsp dried oregano
- Salt and pepper to taste

For the Grilled Chicken:
- 4 boneless, skinless chicken breasts
- 1 tbsp olive oil
- 1 tsp dried thyme
- 1/2 tsp garlic powder
- Salt and pepper to taste

87. Grilled chicken with ratatouille

1. In a large skillet, heat the olive oil over medium•high heat. Add the cubed chicken and cook for 5•7 minutes until browned and cooked through. Remove the chicken from the pan and set aside.

2. In the same skillet, sauté the onion for 3•4 minutes until translucent. Add the garlic and cook for 1 minute more.

3. Add the Arborio rice to the skillet and stir to coat with the oil. Cook for 2•3 minutes, stirring frequently, until the rice is lightly toasted.

4. Slowly pour in the chicken broth, 1/2 cup at a time, stirring constantly, until the liquid is absorbed before adding more. Continue this process for 18•20 minutes, until the rice is tender and creamy.

5. Stir in the cooked chicken, frozen peas, carrots, and zucchini. Cook for 5 more minutes until the vegetables are tender.

6. Remove from heat and stir in the Parmesan cheese and chopped parsley. Season with salt and pepper to taste.

7. Serve the chicken and vegetable risotto warm. Garnish with extra parsley if desired.

This risotto is a complete meal with lean protein, complex carbs, and plenty of veggies. The creamy texture and savory flavors make it a satisfying and nutritious dish for active teen boys.

INGREDIENTS

- 4 (6 oz) cod fillets
- 2 tbsp olive oil
- 1 (14.5 oz) can diced tomatoes
- 2 tbsp capers, drained
- 2 garlic cloves, minced
- 1 tsp dried oregano
- 1/4 tsp red pepper flakes (optional)
- Salt and black pepper to taste
- Chopped fresh parsley for garnish

88. Baked cod with tomato and caper sauce

1. Preheat grill to medium•high heat.

2. Brush the portobello mushroom caps all over with the olive oil. Season with a pinch of salt and pepper.

3. Place the mushroom caps gill•side up on the preheated grill. Grill for 4•5 minutes per side, until the mushrooms are tender and juicy.

4. Remove the grilled mushroom caps from the grill and place them gill•side up on a baking sheet or cutting board.

5. Preheat oven to 400°F.

6. Spread about 1/4 cup of marinara or pizza sauce evenly over the top of each grilled mushroom cap.

7. Sprinkle the shredded mozzarella cheese over the sauce, followed by the sliced pepperoni (if using).

8. Top with the grated Parmesan cheese and a sprinkle of dried oregano.

9. Bake the stuffed mushroom caps in the preheated oven for 8•10 minutes, until the cheese is melted and bubbly.

10. Serve the grilled portobello mushroom cap pizzas immediately, garnished with extra oregano if desired.

These grilled portobello pizzas are a fun and healthy twist on traditional pizza. The mushroom caps act as the "crust" and provide a nutritious, low•carb base. This recipe is sure to be a hit with active teen boys!

INGREDIENTS

- 2 acorn squash, halved and seeded
- 1 cup cooked quinoa
- 1 cup diced mushrooms
- 1/2 cup diced onion
- 2 garlic cloves, minced
- 1 tsp ground cumin
- 1 tsp dried oregano
- 1/4 cup chopped walnuts
- 2 tbsp chopped fresh parsley
- 2 tbsp grated Parmesan cheese
- Salt and pepper to taste

89. Quinoa-stuffed acorn squash

INSTRUCTIONS

1. In a large skillet or wok, heat the olive oil over medium•high heat.

2. Add the sliced beef and cook for 3•4 minutes, stirring frequently, until browned on the outside but still pink in the center.

3. Add the sliced bell peppers and onions to the skillet. Cook for 5•7 minutes, stirring occasionally, until the vegetables are tender•crisp.

4. Stir in the minced garlic, chili powder, cumin, oregano, and a pinch of salt and pepper. Cook for 1 minute until fragrant.

5. Remove the beef and vegetable mixture from the heat.

6. Warm the whole wheat tortillas or wraps according to package instructions.

7. To assemble the fajitas, place some of the beef and vegetable mixture into the center of each tortilla. Top with desired toppings like guacamole, salsa, shredded lettuce, diced tomatoes, and a dollop of low•fat sour cream.

8. Fold the sides of the tortilla over the filling and enjoy!

These lean beef and veggie fajitas are packed with protein, fiber, and nutrients to fuel active teen boys. The combination of lean meat, fresh veggies, and whole grains makes it a balanced and satisfying meal.

INGREDIENTS

- 1 lb large shrimp, peeled and deveined
- 1 red bell pepper, cut into 1-inch pieces
- 1 zucchini, cut into 1-inch pieces
- 1 red onion, cut into 1-inch pieces
- 8 oz mushrooms, halved
- 2 tbsp olive oil
- 2 tbsp lemon juice
- 2 garlic cloves, minced
- 1 tsp dried oregano
- 1/2 tsp paprika
- Salt and pepper to taste
- Wooden or metal skewers

90. Grilled shrimp and vegetable skewers

1. Preheat your oven to 325°F (165°C). Line 1•2 baking sheets with parchment paper.

2. Wash the kale and pat it completely dry with paper towels or a clean kitchen towel. Make sure there is no excess moisture on the leaves.

3. Remove the tough stems from the kale leaves and tear or cut the leaves into bite•sized pieces.

4. Place the kale pieces in a large bowl and drizzle with the olive oil. Use your hands to massage the oil evenly over the kale.

5. Sprinkle the kale with the salt and pepper, and any other desired seasonings. Toss to coat.

6. Arrange the seasoned kale pieces in a single layer on the prepared baking sheets, making sure they are not overlapping.

7. Bake for 12•15 minutes, flipping the kale halfway through, until the chips are crispy and lightly browned.

8. Remove the baked kale chips from the oven and let them cool completely on the baking sheets.

9. Once cooled, transfer the kale chips to an airtight container. They will stay crispy for up to 5 days.

These baked kale chips make a delicious and nutritious snack for active teen boys. They're packed with vitamins, minerals, and fiber, and the crunchy texture is super satisfying. Experiment with different seasonings to find their favorite flavor!

INGREDIENTS

- 8 bone-in, skin-on chicken thighs
- 2 tbsp olive oil, divided
- 1 tsp garlic powder
- 1 tsp dried thyme
- 1/2 tsp salt
- 1/4 tsp black pepper
- 1 lb Brussels sprouts, trimmed and halved
- 2 tbsp balsamic vinegar

91. Baked chicken thighs with roasted Brussels sprouts

1. Toast the whole grain bagels until lightly golden brown.

2. Spread each toasted bagel half with about 1•2 tbsp of the reduced•fat cream cheese.

3. Top the cream cheese with slices of smoked salmon, dividing it evenly between the 4 bagel halves.

4. If desired, sprinkle the smoked salmon with capers and thinly sliced red onion.

5. Garnish the bagels with fresh dill sprigs.

6. Season with a pinch of salt and pepper.

7. Serve the whole grain bagels with cream cheese and smoked salmon immediately.

This open•faced bagel makes for a nutrient•dense and satisfying breakfast or snack for teen boys. The whole grain bagel provides complex carbs and fiber, the cream cheese offers protein and healthy fats, and the smoked salmon is a great source of omega•3s.

The optional toppings like capers, red onion, and dill add extra flavor and nutrition. This is a well•balanced meal that will keep teen boys feeling full and energized.

INGREDIENTS

- 2 tbsp olive oil
- 1 onion, diced
- 3 garlic cloves, minced
- 2 carrots, peeled and diced
- 2 celery stalks, diced
- 1 zucchini, diced
- 1 (15 oz) can diced tomatoes
- 4 cups low-sodium vegetable broth
- 1 (15 oz) can kidney beans, rinsed and drained
- 1 (15 oz) can cannellini beans, rinsed and drained
- 2 cups chopped kale or spinach
- 1 tsp dried oregano
- 1 tsp dried basil
- Salt and black pepper to taste
- Grated Parmesan cheese for serving (optional)

92. Vegetable and bean minestrone soup

INSTRUCTIONS

1. In a large pot or Dutch oven, heat the olive oil over medium heat. Add the diced onion and sauté for 3•4 minutes until translucent.

2. Add the minced garlic and sauté for 1 minute until fragrant.

3. Stir in the diced carrots, celery, bell pepper, and zucchini. Cook for 5•7 minutes, stirring occasionally, until the vegetables start to soften.

4. Add the drained and rinsed chickpeas, diced tomatoes, vegetable/chicken broth, thyme, oregano, and smoked paprika. Season with salt and pepper to taste.

5. Bring the stew to a simmer, then reduce heat to medium•low. Let the stew simmer for 20•25 minutes, stirring occasionally, until the vegetables are tender.

6. Taste and adjust seasonings as needed.

7. Serve the vegetable and chickpea stew hot, garnished with chopped parsley if desired. Crusty bread or rolls make a great accompaniment.

This hearty stew is packed with fiber, protein, vitamins, and minerals from the vegetables and chickpeas. It's a nutritious and satisfying meal that will keep active teen boys feeling full and energized.

INGREDIENTS

- 4 (6 oz) salmon fillets
- 1 lb asparagus, trimmed
- 2 tbsp olive oil, divided
- 1 tsp lemon zest
- 2 tbsp lemon juice
- 1 tsp Dijon mustard
- 1 garlic clove, minced
- 1/4 tsp salt
- 1/4 tsp black pepper

93. Grilled salmon with asparagus

INSTRUCTIONS

1. Preheat grill or grill pan to medium•high heat.

2. Brush the chicken breasts with 1 tbsp of the olive oil and season with the garlic powder, oregano, salt, and pepper.

3. Grill the chicken for 5•7 minutes per side, until cooked through and no longer pink in the center. Let the chicken rest for 5 minutes, then slice or chop it into bite•sized pieces.

4. Warm the whole wheat tortillas or wraps according to package instructions.

5. In a large bowl, toss the chopped romaine lettuce with the remaining 1 tbsp of olive oil and the Caesar dressing.

6. Divide the dressed Caesar salad evenly among the warmed tortillas/wraps.

7. Top the salad with the grilled chicken pieces and sprinkle with the shredded Parmesan cheese.

8. Fold the bottom of the wrap up over the filling, then fold in the sides and continue rolling up tightly to create a wrap.

9. Serve the grilled chicken Caesar wraps immediately.

These wraps are a great balance of lean protein, veggies, and healthy fats to fuel active teen boys. The grilled chicken, crisp romaine, and creamy Caesar dressing make for a delicious and satisfying meal.

INGREDIENTS

- 1 block (14 oz) extra-firm tofu, pressed and cubed
- 2 tbsp olive oil, divided
- 1 onion, diced
- 3 garlic cloves, minced
- 1 tbsp grated fresh ginger
- 2 tsp curry powder
- 1 tsp ground cumin
- 1/2 tsp ground turmeric
- 1/4 tsp cayenne pepper (optional)
- 1 red bell pepper, sliced
- 1 cup cauliflower florets
- 1 cup broccoli florets
- 1 (13.5 oz) can coconut milk
- 1 cup low-sodium vegetable broth
- 2 tbsp tomato paste
- 1 tsp grated lime zest
- 2 tbsp fresh lime juice
- Salt and black pepper to taste
- Chopped cilantro for garnish

94. Baked tofu and vegetable curry

INSTRUCTIONS

1. Preheat oven to 375°F.

2. In a large skillet, cook the ground turkey over medium•high heat until browned and cooked through, 5•7 minutes. Drain any excess fat.

3. Add the olive oil, onion, carrots, celery, and garlic to the skillet. Sauté for 5•7 minutes until the vegetables are tender.

4. Stir in the frozen peas, corn, tomato paste, thyme, rosemary, and season with salt and pepper to taste. Cook for 2•3 minutes.

5. Transfer the turkey and vegetable mixture to a 9x13 inch baking dish.

6. Spread the mashed potatoes evenly over the top of the filling. Sprinkle the shredded cheddar cheese over the potatoes.

7. Bake the shepherd's pie for 25•30 minutes, until the potatoes are lightly browned and the filling is bubbling.

8. Let the shepherd's pie cool for 5•10 minutes before serving.

This turkey and vegetable shepherd's pie is a complete meal in one dish. The lean protein, veggies, and creamy mashed potato topping make it a hearty and satisfying option for active teen boys. Serve with a side salad for a balanced meal.

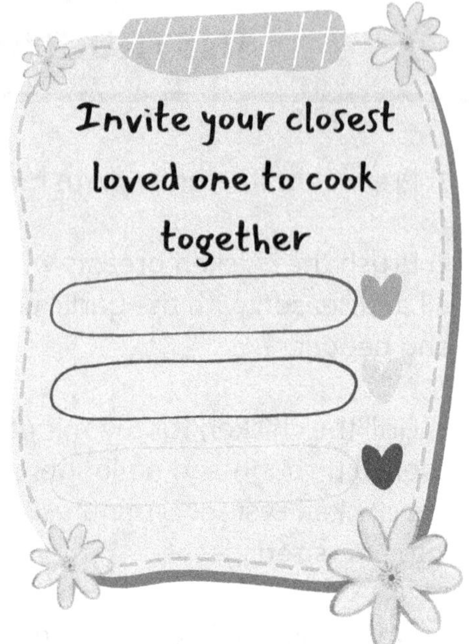

INGREDIENTS

- 1 lb ground turkey
- 2 tbsp sesame oil, divided
- 3 garlic cloves, minced
- 1 tbsp grated fresh ginger
- 1 red bell pepper, sliced
- 1 cup broccoli florets
- 1 cup sliced mushrooms
- 1 cup snow peas or snap peas
- 2 tbsp low-sodium soy sauce
- 1 tbsp rice vinegar
- 1 tsp honey
- 1/4 tsp red pepper flakes (optional)
- Salt and pepper to taste
- Cooked brown rice, for serving

95. Turkey and vegetable stir-fry

INSTRUCTIONS

1. Preheat your oven to 375°F (190°C). Lightly grease a baking sheet or casserole dish.

2. Slice the zucchinis in half lengthwise and use a spoon to scoop out the insides, leaving about 1/4 inch of zucchini flesh along the sides and bottom. Chop the scooped out zucchini flesh.

3. In a skillet over medium heat, cook the ground turkey or beef until browned and crumbled, 5•7 minutes. Drain any excess fat.

4. Add the diced onion and minced garlic to the skillet. Sauté for 2•3 minutes until the onion is translucent.

5. Stir in the chopped zucchini flesh, diced tomatoes, oregano, basil, salt, and pepper. Cook for 5 more minutes.

6. Arrange the zucchini halves cut•side up on the prepared baking sheet or in the casserole dish.

7. Spoon the turkey/beef and vegetable mixture evenly into the zucchini boats.

8. Top each stuffed zucchini boat with shredded mozzarella and grated Parmesan cheese.

9. Bake for 20•25 minutes, until the zucchini is tender and the cheese is melted and bubbly.

10. Serve the baked zucchini boats warm. Enjoy!

These zucchini boats are a great low•carb, veggie•packed meal or side dish. The combination of lean protein, melty cheese, and fresh herbs makes them super flavorful.

INGREDIENTS

- 4 mackerel fillets (about 1 lb total)
- 2 tbsp olive oil, plus more for drizzling
- 1 tsp smoked paprika
- 1 tsp dried oregano
- Salt and pepper to taste
- 2 bell peppers (mix of red, yellow, and/or orange), sliced
- 2 tbsp balsamic vinegar
- 2 tbsp chopped fresh parsley

96. Grilled mackerel with roasted bell peppers

1. Bring a large pot of salted water to a boil. Cook the whole grain pasta according to package instructions until al dente. Drain and set aside.

2. Preheat grill or grill pan to medium•high heat. Brush the chicken breasts with 1 tbsp of the olive oil and season with the garlic powder, salt, and pepper.

3. Grill the chicken for 5•7 minutes per side, until cooked through. Let the chicken rest for 5 minutes, then slice or chop it into bite•sized pieces.

4. In a food processor, combine the basil, 2 cloves of garlic, pine nuts/walnuts, and Parmesan cheese. Pulse until finely chopped.

5. With the food processor running, slowly drizzle in the remaining 2 tbsp of olive oil. Add 1•2 tbsp of water as needed to reach your desired pesto consistency.

6. In a large bowl, toss the cooked whole grain pasta with the prepared pesto until evenly coated.

7. Fold the grilled chicken pieces into the pesto pasta.

8. Serve the whole grain pasta with pesto and grilled chicken warm. Garnish with extra Parmesan cheese if desired.

This dish provides a great balance of lean protein, complex carbs, healthy fats, and fresh flavors to fuel active teen boys. The whole grain pasta, pesto, and grilled chicken make it a satisfying and nutritious meal.

INGREDIENTS

- 1 large eggplant, sliced lengthwise into 1/4-inch thick slices
- 2 tbsp olive oil, plus more for brushing
- 1 cup part-skim ricotta cheese
- 1 cup chopped fresh spinach
- 1/4 cup grated Parmesan cheese
- 1 garlic clove, minced
- 1 tsp dried oregano
- 1/4 tsp red pepper flakes (optional)
- Salt and black pepper to taste
- 1 cup marinara sauce
- 1/2 cup shredded mozzarella cheese

97. Baked eggplant rolls with ricotta and spinach

1. Preheat your oven to 400°F (200°C) or prepare a grill for medium•high heat.

2. Tear off 4 large sheets of heavy•duty aluminum foil, about 12x18 inches each.

3. In a large bowl, toss the chopped vegetables with the olive oil, lemon juice, dill, garlic powder, salt, and pepper until evenly coated.

4. Divide the seasoned vegetables evenly onto the center of each foil sheet.

5. Place one fish fillet on top of the vegetables on each foil sheet.

6. Fold the foil over the fish and vegetables, and crimp the edges to seal the packets completely.

7. If baking, place the foil packets on a baking sheet and bake for 18•22 minutes, until the fish is cooked through and flakes easily with a fork.

8. If grilling, place the foil packets directly on the grill grates and grill for 15•18 minutes, flipping halfway through, until the fish is cooked.

9. Carefully open the foil packets and serve the fish and vegetables immediately, with lemon wedges on the side.

These foil packet meals are easy to prepare, cook quickly, and contain a balance of lean protein, vegetables, and healthy fats to fuel active teen boys. The sealed packets also help retain moisture and flavor. Enjoy!

INGREDIENTS

- 1 cup brown or green lentils, rinsed
- 4 cups vegetable broth
- 1 tbsp olive oil
- 1 onion, diced
- 3 carrots, peeled and diced
- 3 celery stalks, diced
- 3 garlic cloves, minced
- 1 tsp dried thyme
- 1 tsp dried rosemary
- 1 tsp Worcestershire sauce (use vegan if desired)
- Salt and pepper to taste
- 4 cups mashed potatoes (about 6-8 medium potatoes)
- 2 tbsp butter or vegan butter

98. Lentil and vegetable shepherd's pie

1. Preheat grill or grill pan to medium•high heat.

2. In a large bowl, toss the sliced zucchini, squash, bell pepper, and onion with the olive oil. Season with salt and pepper.

3. Grill the vegetables for 2•3 minutes per side, until charred and tender. Transfer to a platter.

4. In a food processor, combine the drained chickpeas, garlic, tahini, lemon juice, water, cumin, and paprika. Blend until smooth and creamy. Season with salt and pepper to taste.

5. Transfer the hummus to a serving bowl and place it in the center of the platter with the grilled vegetables arranged around it.

6. Serve the grilled vegetable and hummus platter immediately, with pita bread or whole grain crackers on the side.

This platter provides a variety of nutrient•dense vegetables paired with a protein•rich hummus dip. The grilled veggies add a delicious smoky flavor, while the creamy hummus offers healthy fats and fiber. It's a great snack or appetizer that teen boys are sure to enjoy.

INGREDIENTS

- 1 lb lean steak (such as sirloin, flank or skirt steak)
- 2 tbsp olive oil, divided
- 1 tsp garlic powder
- 1 tsp dried oregano
- Salt and pepper to taste
- 2 bell peppers, sliced
- 1 zucchini, sliced into rounds
- 1 red onion, sliced into rings
- 2 cups mushrooms, halved
- 1 tbsp balsamic vinegar

99. Grilled lean steak with grilled vegetables

INSTRUCTIONS

1. In a large pot or Dutch oven, heat the olive oil over medium•high heat. Add the beef cubes and brown on all sides, about 5 minutes total. Remove the beef from the pot and set aside.

2. Add the diced onion, carrots, and celery to the pot. Sauté for 5•7 minutes until the vegetables start to soften.

3. Stir in the minced garlic and cook for 1 minute until fragrant.

4. Pour in the beef or chicken broth and add the diced tomatoes, bay leaves, thyme, and oregano. Bring the soup to a simmer.

5. Return the browned beef cubes to the pot. Reduce heat to medium•low and let the soup simmer for 45•60 minutes, until the beef is very tender.

6. Stir in the frozen green beans and peas. Cook for 5•10 more minutes until the vegetables are heated through.

7. Taste the soup and season with salt and pepper as needed.

8. Ladle the beef and vegetable soup into bowls and garnish with chopped parsley if desired.

This hearty soup is packed with lean protein, fiber, and nutrients to fuel active teen boys. The combination of tender beef, fresh veggies, and savory broth makes it a satisfying and comforting meal.

INGREDIENTS

- 1 lb cod fillets
- 2 tbsp olive oil
- 2 tbsp lemon juice
- 2 garlic cloves, minced
- 1 tsp dried oregano
- 1 tsp dried basil
- 1/2 tsp dried thyme
- 1/4 tsp crushed red pepper flakes (optional)
- Salt and pepper to taste
- 2 tbsp chopped fresh parsley

100. Baked cod with Mediterranean herbs

INSTRUCTIONS

1. Preheat your oven to 400°F (200°C). Line a large baking sheet with parchment paper.

2. In a large bowl, toss the carrot fry shapes with the olive oil, garlic powder, paprika, salt, and pepper until the carrots are evenly coated.

3. Spread the seasoned carrot fries in a single layer on the prepared baking sheet, making sure they are not overlapping.

4. Bake for 20•25 minutes, flipping the fries halfway through, until they are tender and lightly browned on the edges.

5. Remove the baked carrot fries from the oven and let them cool for 5 minutes before serving.

Tips:
• For extra crispiness, broil the fries for 2•3 minutes at the end.
• Try different seasoning blends like chili powder, cumin, or Cajun spice.
• Serve the baked carrot fries as a healthy snack or side dish.

These baked carrot fries are a nutritious and delicious alternative to traditional potato fries. Carrots are packed with vitamins, minerals, and fiber, making them a great choice for active teen boys. The crispy exterior and soft interior will have them coming back for more!

INGREDIENTS

- 2 tbsp olive oil
- 1 onion, diced
- 3 garlic cloves, minced
- 1 tsp ground cumin
- 1 tsp ground coriander
- 1 tsp paprika
- 1/2 tsp ground cinnamon
- 1/4 tsp cayenne pepper (or to taste)
- 1 (15oz) can chickpeas, drained and rinsed
- 1 (14oz) can diced tomatoes
- 1 cup vegetable broth
- 2 medium carrots, peeled and sliced
- 1 medium zucchini, sliced
- 1 red bell pepper, sliced
- 1 cup cauliflower florets
- 1 cup green beans, trimmed and cut into 1-inch pieces
- Salt and pepper to taste
- Chopped fresh parsley for garnish

101. Vegetable and chickpea tagine

1. Cook the brown or wild rice according to package instructions. Set aside.

2. In a small bowl, whisk together all the ingredients for the teriyaki sauce. Set aside.

3. Season the chicken breasts with salt and pepper.

4. Heat the 1 tbsp of sesame oil in a large skillet or grill pan over medium•high heat. Add the chicken and cook for 5•7 minutes per side, until cooked through.

5. Transfer the cooked chicken to a cutting board and let rest for 5 minutes. Then slice or shred the chicken.

6. Pour the teriyaki sauce into the skillet and bring to a simmer. Add the shredded chicken and toss to coat.

7. To assemble the rice bowls, divide the cooked rice among 4 serving bowls. Top each with the teriyaki chicken, shredded carrots, shredded red cabbage, and sliced green onions.

8. Sprinkle the toasted sesame seeds over the top of each rice bowl.

9. Serve the whole grain rice bowls with teriyaki chicken immediately.

This meal provides a balance of whole grains, lean protein, vegetables, and flavorful teriyaki sauce. It's a nutritious and satisfying option that teen boys are sure to enjoy.

INGREDIENTS

Roasted Vegetable Quinoa:
- 1 cup uncooked quinoa, rinsed
- 2 cups vegetable or chicken broth
- 1 red bell pepper, diced
- 1 zucchini, diced
- 1 red onion, diced
- 2 tbsp olive oil
- 1 tsp dried oregano
- Salt and pepper to taste

Grilled Chicken:
- 4 boneless, skinless chicken breasts
- 2 tbsp olive oil
- 1 tsp garlic powder
- 1 tsp paprika
- Salt and pepper to taste

INSTRUCTIONS

1. Preheat your oven to 375°F (190°C). Grease a 9x5 inch loaf pan.

2. In a large bowl, combine the cooked lentils, onion, mushrooms, carrots, cooked quinoa, breadcrumbs, eggs, tomato paste, thyme, garlic powder, smoked paprika, salt, and pepper. Mix well until fully incorporated.

3. Transfer the lentil and vegetable mixture to the prepared loaf pan, pressing it down firmly.

4. In a small bowl, whisk together the ingredients for the glaze. Spread the glaze evenly over the top of the loaf.

5. Bake for 45•55 minutes, until the loaf is firm and the top is lightly browned.

6. Let the lentil and vegetable loaf cool in the pan for 10 minutes before slicing and serving.

This meatless loaf is packed with plant•based protein from the lentils and quinoa, as well as plenty of fiber and nutrients from the vegetables. The glaze adds a nice sweet and tangy flavor. Serve it with roasted potatoes, a fresh salad, or your teen's favorite sides for a complete and satisfying meal.

INGREDIENTS

- 1 lb ground turkey
- 1 cup fresh spinach, finely chopped
- 1/2 cup breadcrumbs
- 1/4 cup grated Parmesan cheese
- 1 egg
- 2 garlic cloves, minced
- 1 tsp dried oregano
- 1/2 tsp salt
- 1/4 tsp black pepper

1. If using wooden skewers, soak them in water for 30 minutes to prevent burning.

2. In a large bowl, combine the shrimp, zucchini, bell pepper, onion, and mushrooms. Drizzle with the olive oil and lemon juice, then sprinkle with the oregano, garlic powder, salt, and pepper. Toss to coat everything evenly.

3. Thread the shrimp and vegetables onto the skewers, alternating the ingredients.

4. Preheat grill or grill pan to medium•high heat.

5. Grill the skewers for 2•3 minutes per side, until the shrimp are opaque and the vegetables are tender•crisp.

6. Serve the grilled shrimp and vegetable skewers immediately.

Tips:
• For extra flavor, marinate the shrimp and vegetables for 30 minutes to 1 hour before grilling.
• Try different vegetable combinations like cherry tomatoes, asparagus, or pineapple.
• Serve the skewers over a bed of quinoa or brown rice for a more substantial meal.

These grilled shrimp and veggie skewers are a great source of lean protein, fiber, and nutrients. The bright flavors and fun presentation make them an appealing and healthy option for active teen boys.

INGREDIENTS

Tomato Salad:
- 2 cups cherry or grape tomatoes, halved
- 1/2 red onion, thinly sliced
- 1 tbsp olive oil
- 1 tbsp red wine vinegar
- 1 tbsp chopped fresh basil
- Salt and pepper to taste

Grilled Sardines:
- 8 fresh sardine fillets
- 2 tbsp olive oil
- 1 tsp lemon zest
- 1 tbsp lemon juice
- 2 garlic cloves, minced
- Salt and pepper to taste

1. Preheat your oven to 375°F (190°C). Lightly grease a baking sheet.

2. Remove the stems from the mushrooms and finely chop them. Set the mushroom caps aside.

3. In a skillet over medium heat, heat the olive oil. Add the chopped mushroom stems, ground turkey, and minced garlic. Cook for 5•7 minutes, breaking up the turkey as it cooks, until the turkey is browned and cooked through.

4. Remove the skillet from heat and stir in the chopped spinach, Parmesan cheese, breadcrumbs, and oregano. Season with salt and pepper to taste.

5. Spoon the turkey and spinach mixture evenly into the mushroom caps, packing it in gently.

6. Arrange the stuffed mushrooms on the prepared baking sheet.

7. Bake for 12•15 minutes, until the mushrooms are tender and the filling is hot.

8. Serve the turkey and spinach stuffed mushrooms warm.

These stuffed mushrooms make a great protein•packed and veggie•filled snack or appetizer for teen boys. The combination of savory turkey, fresh spinach, and melty cheese is sure to be a hit. You can also make them ahead of time and bake right before serving.

INGREDIENTS

- 8 oz tempeh, cut into 1-inch cubes
- 2 cups broccoli florets
- 1 cup cooked brown rice
- 2 tbsp soy sauce or tamari
- 1 tbsp sesame oil
- 1 tsp garlic powder
- 1/2 tsp ground ginger
- Salt and pepper to taste

105. Baked tempeh with broccoli and brown rice

INSTRUCTIONS

1. Preheat your oven to 400°F (200°C). Line a large baking sheet with parchment paper.

2. In a large bowl, toss the cut butternut squash fries with the olive oil, garlic powder, paprika, salt, and pepper until the fries are evenly coated.

3. Spread the seasoned butternut squash fries in a single layer on the prepared baking sheet, making sure they are not overlapping.

4. Bake for 25•30 minutes, flipping the fries halfway through, until they are tender and lightly browned on the edges.

5. Remove the baked butternut squash fries from the oven and let them cool for 5 minutes before serving.

Tips:
• For extra crispiness, broil the fries for 2•3 minutes at the end.
• Try different seasoning blends like chili powder, cumin, or cajun spice.
• Serve the baked butternut squash fries as a healthy snack or side dish.

These baked butternut squash fries are a nutritious and delicious alternative to traditional potato fries. Butternut squash is packed with vitamins, minerals, and fiber, making it a great choice for active teen boys. The sweet, caramelized flavor and crispy texture will have them coming back for more!

INGREDIENTS

- 8-10 whole grain tortillas
- 1 can (15 oz) black beans, rinsed and drained
- 1 can (15 oz) pinto beans, rinsed and drained
- 2 cups diced bell peppers (mix of red, yellow, orange)
- 1 cup diced onion
- 2 cups chopped spinach or kale
- 2 tsp ground cumin
- 1 tsp chili powder
- 1/2 tsp garlic powder
- Salt and pepper to taste
- 1 can (15 oz) enchilada sauce
- 1 cup shredded cheddar or Monterey Jack cheese

INSTRUCTIONS

1. In a medium bowl, mash the black beans with a fork or potato masher. Stir in the chili powder, cumin, salt, and pepper.

2. Lay the whole grain tortillas out on a flat surface. Spread the seasoned black bean mixture evenly over half of each tortilla.

3. Sprinkle the shredded cheese over the black beans.

4. Fold the other half of the tortilla over the filling to create a half•moon shape.

5. Heat the olive oil in a large skillet or griddle over medium heat.

6. Working in batches if needed, add the quesadillas to the hot skillet. Cook for 2•3 minutes per side, until the tortillas are lightly golden brown and the cheese is melted.

7. Remove the quesadillas from the heat and cut each one in half.

8. Serve the whole grain tortilla bean and cheese quesadillas warm, with salsa, guacamole, or sour cream on the side if desired.

These quesadillas are a great source of protein, fiber, and complex carbs to fuel active teen boys. The whole grain tortillas, black beans, and melty cheese make for a satisfying and nutritious meal or snack.

INGREDIENTS

- 14 oz extra-firm tofu, cut into 1-inch cubes
- 1 red bell pepper, cut into 1-inch pieces
- 1 yellow bell pepper, cut into 1-inch pieces
- 1 zucchini, cut into 1-inch slices
- 1 red onion, cut into 1-inch pieces
- 8 oz mushrooms, halved
- 2 tbsp olive oil
- 2 tbsp soy sauce or tamari
- 1 tsp garlic powder
- 1 tsp dried oregano
- Salt and pepper to taste
- Wooden or metal skewers

107. Grilled tofu and vegetable kebabs

INSTRUCTIONS

1. Cook the brown rice according to package instructions. Set aside.

2. In a small bowl, combine the soy sauce, rice vinegar, and sesame oil. Set aside.

3. Heat the olive oil in a large skillet or wok over high heat. Add the chicken and stir•fry for 4•5 minutes until lightly browned.

4. Add the minced garlic and grated ginger to the skillet. Stir•fry for 1 minute until fragrant.

5. Add the sliced bell pepper, broccoli, snow/snap peas, and mushrooms to the skillet. Stir•fry for 5•7 minutes until the vegetables are tender•crisp.

6. Pour the soy sauce mixture into the skillet and toss everything together. Cook for 2•3 more minutes until the sauce has thickened slightly.

7. Remove from heat and stir in the sliced green onions. Season with salt and pepper to taste.

8. Serve the chicken and vegetable stir•fry immediately over the cooked brown rice.

This stir•fry is packed with lean protein, fiber, vitamins, and minerals to fuel active teen boys. The combination of tender chicken, fresh veggies, and nutty brown rice makes it a satisfying and nutritious meal.

INGREDIENTS

- 4 boneless, skinless chicken breasts
- 1 whole head of garlic
- 2 tbsp olive oil, divided
- 1 tsp dried thyme
- 1 tsp dried rosemary
- Salt and pepper to taste

INSTRUCTIONS

1. Pat the tuna steaks dry with paper towels and brush both sides with the olive oil. Season generously with salt and pepper.

2. Preheat grill or grill pan to medium•high heat.

3. Grill the tuna steaks for 2•3 minutes per side, depending on thickness, until the outside is lightly charred but the inside is still pink and tender.

4. Transfer the grilled tuna steaks to a plate and drizzle with the lemon juice.

5. Serve the grilled tuna steaks immediately, while hot. They pair well with grilled vegetables, rice, or a fresh salad.

The key is not to overcook the tuna • you want it to be seared on the outside but still rare to medium•rare in the center. Enjoy your fresh and flavorful grilled tuna steak!

INGREDIENTS

- 1 cup dry brown or green lentils, rinsed
- 3 cups vegetable broth
- 1 tbsp olive oil
- 1 onion, diced
- 2 carrots, peeled and grated
- 2 celery stalks, diced
- 3 garlic cloves, minced
- 1 cup cooked quinoa
- 1 cup breadcrumbs (use gluten-free if needed)
- 2 eggs, lightly beaten (or 2 flax eggs for vegan)
- 2 tbsp tomato paste
- 1 tsp dried thyme
- 1 tsp dried oregano
- Salt and pepper to taste

For the Glaze:
- 1/4 cup ketchup or tomato sauce
- 2 tbsp maple syrup
- 1 tbsp Dijon mustard

109. Lentil and vegetable loaf

INSTRUCTIONS

1. In a large skillet, heat the olive oil over medium heat. Add the diced bell peppers, mushrooms, and onion. Sauté for 5•7 minutes until the vegetables are tender.

2. Add the minced garlic and crumbled tofu to the skillet. Stir to combine.

3. Sprinkle the nutritional yeast, turmeric, oregano, and cumin over the tofu and vegetables. Season with salt and pepper.

4. Stir the mixture frequently and cook for 5•7 more minutes, until the tofu is heated through and the flavors have melded.

5. Stir in the chopped baby spinach and cook for 2•3 minutes until the spinach is wilted.

6. Remove the vegetable and tofu scramble from heat. Taste and adjust seasonings as needed.

7. Serve the scramble warm, with hot sauce on the side if desired. It's delicious on its own or with whole grain toast, roasted potatoes, or avocado.

This protein•packed, veggie•loaded scramble is a great meatless option for active teen boys. The tofu provides plant•based protein, while the colorful vegetables offer fiber, vitamins, and minerals. It's a nutritious and satisfying breakfast or brunch dish.

INGREDIENTS

- 4 trout fillets (about 6 oz each)
- 2 tbsp olive oil, divided
- 1 tsp lemon zest
- 1 tbsp lemon juice
- 1 tsp dried dill
- Salt and pepper to taste
- 4 cups fresh spinach leaves
- 2 garlic cloves, minced
- 1 tbsp water

INSTRUCTIONS

1. Preheat your oven to 400°F (200°C). Line two baking sheets with parchment paper.

2. In a large bowl, toss the parsnip slices with the olive oil, salt, and pepper until evenly coated.

3. Arrange the parsnip slices in a single layer on the prepared baking sheets, making sure they are not overlapping.

4. Bake for 15•20 minutes, flipping the chips halfway through, until they are golden brown and crispy.

5. Keep a close eye on the chips towards the end to prevent burning. The thinner slices may cook faster than the thicker ones.

6. Remove the baked parsnip chips from the oven and let them cool on the baking sheets for a few minutes before serving.

Tips:
• For extra crispiness, you can soak the parsnip slices in cold water for 30 minutes before patting them dry and tossing with the oil and seasonings.
• Try experimenting with different seasonings, such as garlic powder, paprika, or rosemary.
• Enjoy the baked parsnip chips as a healthy snack or side dish.

INGREDIENTS

- 1 lb boneless, skinless chicken tenders
- 1 cup cooked chickpeas (or 1 (15oz) can, drained and rinsed)
- 1/4 cup fresh parsley, chopped
- 2 garlic cloves, minced
- 1 tsp ground cumin
- 1 tsp ground coriander
- 1/2 tsp baking soda
- 1/4 tsp cayenne pepper (optional)
- Salt and pepper to taste
- 1 egg, beaten
- 1 cup panko breadcrumbs

III. Baked falafel-crusted chicken tenders

INSTRUCTIONS

1. Preheat your grill or grill pan to medium•high heat.

2. Slice the vegetables into long, thin strips. Toss them with a bit of olive oil, salt, and pepper.

3. Grill the vegetables for 5•7 minutes per side, until they are tender and slightly charred.

4. Spread about 1/4 cup of hummus onto each whole grain wrap.

5. Top the hummus with the grilled vegetables, spinach/arugula, and feta cheese (if using).

6. Fold the wrap tightly and cut in half diagonally to serve.

Why this is great for teen boys:
• Whole grains provide complex carbs and fiber to keep them full and energized.
• Grilled vegetables add important vitamins, minerals, and antioxidants.
• Hummus provides protein and healthy fats to support growth and development.
• The wrap format is easy to eat on•the•go, perfect for busy teens.
• The flavors and textures make it a satisfying and delicious meal.

Encourage your teen boys to customize the wrap with their favorite veggies or other toppings. This is a nutritious and portable option they're sure to enjoy!

INGREDIENTS

- 1 tbsp olive oil
- 1 onion, diced
- 3 carrots, peeled and diced
- 3 celery stalks, diced
- 3 garlic cloves, minced
- 1 cup pearl barley, rinsed
- 6 cups low-sodium vegetable broth
- 1 (14.5 oz) can diced tomatoes
- 2 cups chopped kale or spinach
- 1 tsp dried thyme
- 1 tsp dried oregano
- Salt and pepper to taste
- Chopped parsley for garnish (optional)

112. Vegetable and barley soup

1. Preheat your oven to 375°F (190°C).

2. In a large saucepan, combine the lentils and vegetable broth. Bring to a boil, then reduce heat and simmer for 20•25 minutes, until the lentils are tender. Drain any excess liquid.

3. In a large skillet, heat the olive oil over medium heat. Add the onion, carrots, celery, and garlic. Sauté for 5•7 minutes, until the vegetables are softened.

4. Add the cooked lentils, thyme, rosemary, Worcestershire sauce, and season with salt and pepper to taste. Stir to combine.

5. Transfer the lentil and vegetable mixture to a 9x13 inch baking dish.

6. Spread the mashed potatoes evenly over the top of the lentil mixture. If using, sprinkle the shredded cheddar cheese over the potatoes.

7. Bake for 25•30 minutes, until the potatoes are lightly browned and the filling is bubbling.

8. Let the shepherd's pie cool for 5•10 minutes before serving.

Why this is great for teen boys:
• Lentils provide a plant•based source of protein, fiber, and complex carbs to keep them full and energized.
• The vegetables add important vitamins, minerals, and antioxidants.
• The mashed potato topping is comforting and satisfying.
• The flavors and textures make it a delicious and hearty meal.

INGREDIENTS

- 1 lb lean pork tenderloin
- 2 tbsp olive oil
- 2 tsp garlic powder
- 1 tsp dried thyme
- Salt and pepper to taste
- 3-4 ripe peaches, halved and pitted
- 1 tbsp honey
- 1 tbsp balsamic vinegar

113. Grilled lean pork tenderloin with grilled peaches

1. Preheat grill or grill pan to medium•high heat.

2. In a large bowl, toss the chicken, bell peppers, onion, and mushrooms with the olive oil and fajita seasoning until well coated.

3. Grill the chicken for 6•8 minutes per side, until cooked through. Grill the vegetables for 5•7 minutes, stirring occasionally, until tender and slightly charred.

4. Remove the chicken and vegetables from the grill and let rest for a few minutes. Slice the chicken into strips.

5. Assemble the fajita bowls by dividing the brown rice, black beans, grilled chicken, and grilled vegetables among 4 bowls.

6. Top each bowl with shredded cheddar cheese, salsa, and a dollop of sour cream (if using).

Why this is great for teen boys:
• Grilled chicken and vegetables provide lean protein, fiber, and important vitamins and minerals.
• Brown rice and black beans offer complex carbs, fiber, and plant•based protein to keep them full and energized.
• The fajita flavors and customizable toppings make it a tasty and satisfying meal.
• The bowl format is easy to eat and portable, perfect for busy teens.

Encourage your teen boys to customize their bowls with their favorite toppings or sauces. This is a nutritious and delicious meal they're sure to enjoy!

INGREDIENTS

- 4 (6 oz) cod fillets
- 2 tbsp olive oil
- Salt and pepper to taste
- 2 tbsp unsalted butter
- 2 tbsp capers, drained and rinsed
- 2 tbsp freshly squeezed lemon juice
- 2 tbsp chopped fresh parsley
- Lemon wedges for serving

114. Baked cod with lemon and caper sauce

INSTRUCTIONS

1. Preheat your oven to 400°F (200°C). Line a baking sheet with parchment paper.

2. In a large bowl, combine the ground turkey, chopped vegetables, breadcrumbs, egg, Parmesan, garlic, oregano, salt, and pepper. Mix until well incorporated.

3. Roll the mixture into 1•inch meatballs and place them on the prepared baking sheet.

4. Bake the meatballs for 18•20 minutes, until cooked through and lightly browned.

5. While the meatballs are baking, cook the whole grain pasta according to package instructions. Drain and set aside.

6. In a large saucepan, heat the marinara sauce over medium heat until warmed through.

7. Add the cooked meatballs to the marinara sauce and gently stir to coat.

8. Serve the turkey and vegetable meatballs over the cooked whole grain pasta.

Why this is great for teen boys:
• Ground turkey provides lean protein to support growth and development.
• The added vegetables boost the nutrient content and fiber intake.
• Whole grain pasta offers complex carbs and fiber to keep them full and energized.
• The familiar flavors of meatballs and marinara sauce make it a satisfying and delicious meal.
• This dish is easy to prepare and can be made in larger batches for leftovers.

INGREDIENTS

- 6 bell peppers (mix of red, yellow, and orange)
- 1 lb ground turkey
- 1 cup cooked brown rice
- 1 cup diced onion
- 1 cup diced zucchini
- 1 cup diced tomatoes
- 2 garlic cloves, minced
- 1 tsp dried oregano
- 1 tsp dried basil
- Salt and pepper to taste
- 1 cup shredded mozzarella cheese

INSTRUCTIONS

1. Preheat your oven to 400°F (200°C). Line a baking sheet with parchment paper.

2. Pat the drained and rinsed chickpeas dry with paper towels to remove any excess moisture.

3. In a medium bowl, toss the chickpeas with the olive oil, paprika, garlic powder, onion powder, salt, and black pepper until they are evenly coated.

4. Spread the seasoned chickpeas in a single layer on the prepared baking sheet.

5. Bake for 20•25 minutes, stirring halfway, until the chickpeas are crispy and golden brown.

6. Remove the baked chickpeas from the oven and let them cool for a few minutes before serving.

Why this is great for teen boys:
• Chickpeas are a great source of plant•based protein, fiber, and complex carbs to keep them full and energized.
• The baked, crispy texture makes them a satisfying and crunchy snack.
• The flavorful seasoning adds taste appeal and variety.
• Chickpeas are a versatile and portable snack that teen boys can easily grab and enjoy.

Encourage your teen boys to experiment with different seasonings, such as chili powder, cumin, or cajun seasoning, to find their favorite flavor profile. These baked crispy chickpeas make a nutritious and delicious snack that teen boys are sure to love!

INGREDIENTS

For the Chicken:
- 4 boneless, skinless chicken breasts
- 2 tbsp olive oil
- 1 tsp dried oregano
- 1 tsp garlic powder
- Salt and pepper to taste

For the Mediterranean Salad:
- 1 cup cherry tomatoes, halved
- 1 cucumber, diced
- 1/2 red onion, thinly sliced
- 1 cup pitted kalamata olives, halved
- 1/2 cup crumbled feta cheese
- 2 tbsp chopped fresh parsley
- 2 tbsp chopped fresh basil
- 2 tbsp olive oil
- 1 tbsp red wine vinegar
- 1 tsp Dijon mustard
- Salt and pepper to taste

116. Grilled chicken with Mediterranean salad

1. Preheat your grill or grill pan to medium•high heat.

2. Brush the chicken breasts with 1 tbsp of the olive oil and season with the Italian seasoning, salt, and pepper.

3. Grill the chicken for 6•8 minutes per side, until cooked through. Let it rest for a few minutes, then slice or shred the chicken.

4. In a skillet, heat the remaining 1 tbsp of olive oil over medium heat. Add the mixed grilled vegetables and sauté for 5•7 minutes, until tender.

5. Preheat your oven to 400°F (200°C).

6. Spread the marinara sauce evenly over the whole grain pizza crust. Top with the shredded mozzarella cheese, grilled chicken, and sautéed vegetables.

7. Sprinkle the grated Parmesan cheese over the top.

8. Bake the pizza for 12•15 minutes, until the cheese is melted and bubbly.

9. Slice and serve the whole grain pizza hot.

Why this is great for teen boys:
• Whole grain pizza crust provides complex carbs and fiber to keep them full and energized.
• Grilled chicken adds lean protein to support growth and development.
• The variety of grilled vegetables boosts nutrient intake and fiber.
• The familiar flavors of pizza make it a tasty and satisfying meal.
• This dish is easy to prepare and can be customized with their favorite toppings.

INGREDIENTS

- 1 block (14 oz) extra-firm tofu, pressed and cut into 1/2-inch thick slices
- 1 cup panko breadcrumbs
- 1/2 cup grated Parmesan cheese
- 1 tsp dried oregano
- 1/2 tsp garlic powder
- 1/4 tsp salt
- 1/4 tsp black pepper
- 1 egg, beaten
- 1 cup marinara sauce
- 1 cup shredded mozzarella cheese

1. In a large skillet or wok, heat the olive oil over medium heat. Add the onion and sauté for 3•4 minutes until translucent.

2. Add the garlic and ginger, and cook for 1 minute, until fragrant.

3. Stir in the curry powder, cumin, coriander, and turmeric. Cook for 1 minute to toast the spices.

4. Pour in the diced tomatoes and coconut milk. Bring the mixture to a simmer.

5. Add the fish pieces and mixed vegetables to the curry. Gently simmer for 10•12 minutes, until the fish is cooked through and the vegetables are tender.

6. Season the curry with salt and pepper to taste.

7. Serve the fish and vegetable curry over the cooked basmati rice. Garnish with chopped cilantro, if desired.

Why this is great for teen boys:
• White fish provides lean protein to support growth and development.
• The variety of vegetables adds important vitamins, minerals, and fiber.
• The aromatic spices and coconut milk create a flavorful and satisfying curry.
• Basmati rice offers complex carbs to keep them full and energized.
• This dish is easy to prepare and can be made in larger batches for leftovers.

Encourage your teen boys to help prepare the curry and customize it with their favorite vegetables or spices. This fish and vegetable curry is a nutritious and delicious option that teen boys are sure to enjoy.

INGREDIENTS

- 1 cup uncooked quinoa, rinsed
- 2 cups vegetable broth
- 1 tbsp olive oil
- 1 onion, diced
- 3 garlic cloves, minced
- 1 red bell pepper, diced
- 1 jalapeño, seeded and minced (optional)
- 2 cans (15 oz each) black beans, rinsed and drained
- 1 can (15 oz) kidney beans, rinsed and drained
- 1 can (28 oz) diced tomatoes
- 2 tbsp chili powder
- 1 tsp ground cumin
- 1 tsp dried oregano
- 1/2 tsp smoked paprika
- Salt and pepper to taste
- Chopped cilantro for garnish (optional)

1. Preheat your grill or grill pan to medium•high heat.

2. In a small bowl, combine 1 tbsp of the olive oil, garlic powder, onion powder, oregano, salt, and pepper. Rub this seasoning mixture all over the steak.

3. Grill the steak for 4•6 minutes per side, depending on thickness, until it reaches your desired doneness. Let the steak rest for 5 minutes before slicing.

4. Preheat your oven to 400°F (200°C). Line a baking sheet with parchment paper.

5. In a large bowl, toss the mixed vegetables and red onion wedges with the remaining 1 tbsp of olive oil and the minced garlic. Season with salt and pepper.

6. Spread the seasoned vegetables in a single layer on the prepared baking sheet.

7. Roast the vegetables for 20•25 minutes, stirring halfway, until they are tender and lightly browned.

8. Slice the grilled steak and serve it alongside the roasted vegetables.

Why this is great for teen boys:
• Lean steak provides high•quality protein to support muscle growth and development.
• The variety of roasted vegetables adds important vitamins, minerals, and fiber.
• The simple seasoning allows the natural flavors of the steak and vegetables to shine.
• This meal is balanced, satisfying, and easy to prepare.
• Grilling and roasting the components make it a healthy and flavorful option.

INGREDIENTS

- 1 lb large shrimp, peeled and deveined
- 2 tbsp olive oil
- 1 tsp garlic powder
- 1 tsp dried oregano
- Salt and pepper to taste
- 3 medium zucchinis, spiralized or julienned into noodles
- 2 tbsp lemon juice
- 2 tbsp chopped fresh parsley
- 1 tbsp grated Parmesan cheese (optional)

*Thank you for purchasing **"Fatty Liver Cookbook for Men: 115+ Delicious Recipes for Fatty Liver. 60 Day Meal Detox and Cleanse Your Liver."** We are thrilled to be a part of your journey toward better health and wellness.*

This cookbook is designed to provide you with the knowledge and tools necessary to make meaningful dietary changes that support your liver health. With over 115 delicious recipes and a comprehensive 60-day meal plan, you have everything you need to start detoxifying and cleansing your liver today.

Here's what you can look forward to:

- **Delicious and Nutritious Recipes:** *Enjoy a wide variety of meals that are both tasty and beneficial for your liver. From breakfasts that kickstart your day to dinners that aid in healing, you'll find recipes to suit every taste and occasion.*

- **A Structured 60-Day Meal Plan:** *Follow our carefully crafted meal plan to detoxify and cleanse your liver over two months. This plan ensures you get the right balance of nutrients and helps you stay on track with your health goals.*

- **Essential Cooking Tips and Advice:** *Learn how to make healthier food choices, organize your kitchen, and prepare meals efficiently. Our practical tips will make adopting a liver-friendly diet easier and more enjoyable.*

We hope this book becomes a valuable resource for you, providing not just recipes, but a pathway to a healthier lifestyle. Your commitment to improving your liver health is commendable, and we are here to support you every step of the way.

Happy cooking, and here's to your health!

Best regards,

The Fatty Liver Cookbook Team